COMMUNITY BASED NURSING

Foundation for Practice

Ginger Armentrout, EdD, RN
Associate Professor
Leader of Community Health Nursing
School of Nursing
North Carolina Agricultural and Technical
State University
Greensboro, North Carolina

Appleton & Lange
Stamford, Connecticut

Copyright © 1998 by Appleton & Lange
A Simon & Schuster Company

www.appletonlange.com

98 99 00 01 02 / 10 9 8 7 6 5 4 3 2 1

Prentice Hall International (UK) Limited, *London*
Prentice Hall of Australia Pty. Limited, *Sydney*
Prentice Hall of Canada, Inc., *Toronto*
Prentice Hall Hispanoamericana, S.A., *Mexico*
Prentice Hall of India Private Limited, *New Delhi*
Prentice Hall of Japan, Inc., *Tokyo*
Simon & Schuster Asia Pte. Ltd., *Singapore*
Editora Prentice Hall do Brasil Ltda., *Rio de Janeiro*
Prentice Hall, Upper Saddle River, *New Jersey*

Library of Congress Cataloging-in-Publication Data

Armentrout, Ginger H.
    Community based nursing : foundation for practice / Ginger H. Armentrout.
        p.   cm.
    Includes index.
    ISBN 0–8385–1522–3 (alk. paper)
    1. Community health nursing.   I. Title.
    [DNLM: 1. Home Care Services.   WY 115 A728c 1998]
    RT98.A75   1998
    610.73'43—dc21
    DNLM/DLC
    For Library of Congress   97–45780
                                                          CIP

Acquisitions Editor: Patricia Casey
Development Editor: Janet Foltin
Production Editor: Elizabeth C. Ryan
Production Service: Jennsin Services
Designer: Libby Schmitz

ISBN 0-8385-1522-3

9 780838 515228   90000

*This book is dedicated to
my husband, John
our children, Charlie and Bill
my Dad, Fred Halter and the
memory of my mother, Florence
all the students that I taught
and who taught me*

Contents

Preface

Until recently, community health nursing was taught primarily in baccalaureate programs on the undergraduate level. The dramatic changes precipitated by health care reform and managed care have led to the discharge of sicker patients into their homes and into the community resulting in the rapid proliferation of home care agencies and other community based agencies. Associate degree programs nationwide are now introducing community based nursing, not community health nursing, into their curriculums to teach their students to care for clients and their families in this setting.

Hospital nurses are also being affected by the above changes. Many hospitals own home care and other community agencies. As the patient census fluctuates on different units in the hospital, the possibility of temporarily moving excess staff to home care and other community based agencies becomes more and more feasible. Most hospital staff nurses, however, are not prepared to rotate to community based nursing.

This textbook meets the needs of both nursing student and the hospital staff nurse in their pursuit of practice opportunities in the community setting. It is an introduction to the concepts and practice of community based nursing. This book presents a broad overview of the field, speaks to the reader, and is a practical guide.

The book is organized into four parts, namely, an introduction to community based nursing, perspectives of the nurse, knowledge applicable to community based nursing, and specific practice settings of community based nursing. Part I contains two chapters and focuses on the origins and context of community based nursing. A comparison is made between this specialty and hospital, public health, and community health nursing. An overview of the health care system is presented from the perspective of a paradigm shift. Managed care, the financing of health care, and trends that influence nursing care in this environment are discussed. The two chapters in Part II focus on personal and professional perspectives of the nurse. These include the impact of beliefs, skills needed in community based practice, ethical and legal aspects of care, the interdisciplinary team, community resources, and the referral process. Part III contains three chapters and focuses on knowledge applicable to community based nursing that broadens the student's knowledge base to facilitate practicing in the community. This part begins with cultural diversity and continues with the application of the nursing process, critical thinking skills, concepts of public health, and client teaching. Part IV consists of three chapters and contains an in-depth discussion of home visiting, introduces specific practice settings in the community, and concludes with future trends in community based nursing.

An innovative aspect of this text is the critical thinking exercises. These exercises are presented within the chapters, and the student is given the space to complete the exercise before proceeding. The purpose of these critical thinking exercises is twofold. First, they are sequential in nature and stimulate the student to raise questions and come to effective conclusions by synthesizing knowledge for many areas. Second, the student is given the opportunity to comfortably explore beliefs and attitudes that can greatly affect nursing practice. The outcome of these exercises prepares the student for practice in any setting.

This book is unique because it offers students and nurses theoretical and practical content in an integrated manner. The content may be presented in one course or throughout an entire curricculum. *Community Based Nursing: An Integrated Approach* strives to meet the needs of students and nurses working in the community and confronting changes in health care delivery.

Acknowledgments

The completion of this book looks like a delicate spring garden that suddenly came out of nowhere. Of course it really didn't happen that way. So many people, knowingly and unknowingly, provided the conditions that supported its growth every step of the way. My appreciation:

To Jeannie White who sent Ann Finch to the gardener with the seeds

To John Swift, the sales rep for leading me to Sally Barhydt, Editor-in-Chief, who revealed the best season for planting

To Beverly Malone who showed the gardener how to protect the seedlings

To the much needed gentle rain: Kelly Burch, Martha Boschen, Libby Latham, Lori Hodges, and Linda McIntosh

To the clouds, storms, wind, and fertilizer that strengthened the growth

To the seasoned gardeners Rachel Spector and Judy Terry who willingly shared tips

To my good friend Arniece Bowen who continuously nurtured the gardener

To those who willingly shared their expertise: Billie VunCannon, Kentie Roland, Rebecca Moreland, Cyndee Cromer, and Janet Nichols

To Ana Prothro who willingly pulled the weeds and removed any unwanted critters

To Lauren Keller, Trish Casey, and Elisabeth Church, my editors, who provided warm breezes

To Janet Foltin, my development editor, who relentlessly dug in the
    garden, rearranging the plants as needed without missing one
To my husband, John, who provided the sunshine
and
To the students who are free to pick the flowers and enjoy.

COMMUNITY BASED NURSING

Foundation for Practice

I.

INTRODUCTION TO COMMUNITY BASED NURSING

1.

Overview of Nursing in the Community

 exercise 1–1

Describe your impression of nursing practice in the community. How does it differ from hospital nursing?

Nursing practice in the community is primarily focused on health, wellness and prevention. Additional emphasis is placed on disease mgmt. In the hospital, nursing is primarily focused on the treatment of the disease process in an acute phase of an illness.

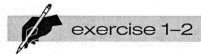

exercise 1–2

As you think about going to a stranger's house to make a nursing visit, list the fears that come up within you.

Environmental
Isolation

Patients are being discharged from the hospital with critical nursing needs, a practice that would have been unthinkable just a few years ago. This has created a dramatic shift of nursing care from acute care settings into the community. There are approximately 2.2 million nurses in the United States today. Eighty-three percent are employed, and two-thirds of them work in the hospital setting. It is estimated that in just five years, less than half of all employed nurses will be working in hospitals (McKinnon, 1997). This makes it quite clear that community based nursing will continue to grow.

WHAT IS COMMUNITY BASED NURSING PRACTICE?

The term **community based nursing** first appeared in the nursing literature about ten years ago, but the term appears more frequently in the last few years. To date, there is not a heading for "community based nursing" in the *Cumulative Index to Nursing & Allied Health Literature* (CINAHL). So, we are dealing with a new label for a very old practice. We will begin with a definition of community based nursing and then we will compare hospital nursing, public health nursing, and community health nursing to community based nursing. As you hear these terms being used by health care professionals, you will understand what they mean.

There are two components to community based nursing. One refers to the setting and the other relates to practice. By definition, the words "community based" means placement in the community.

This usually refers to any setting other than an acute care setting. An acute care institution may include a setting that is non-acute, such as a day care center that provides childcare for the children of employees The day care center would be considered community based because it is separate from the acute setting.

The practice of community based nursing differs from hospital nursing in that, in addition to caring for the client in a particular setting, there is a focus on factors that are a part of the client's life and that affect his health. These include his lifestyle, his family and their relationships with each other, and the impact of the community on the client and his family.

SETTINGS OF NURSING PRACTICE: A COMPARISON

We need to examine what some of the differences are between practicing in the hospital setting and practicing in a community based setting. You know how to practice nursing in the hospital; however, you may not have thought about the many advantages the nurse experiences in that setting or the effect that the setting can have on the patient.

The community based setting requires that you understand aspects of the client's life that will impact your nursing practice. The demands placed on you in the community will vary from the hospital. It is also helpful to know how nursing in the hospital and in the community differ from public health nursing.

Hospital Nursing: The Effect of Institutional Control

In the hospital setting, the health care professional, not the patient, is in control. In fact, the term "patient" implies being the passive recipient of action. We are often unaware of just how powerless the patient may be in the system. Let's review the kinds of experiences that can strip a patient of personal power.

- Admission to the hospital places the patient in a new, strange environment, often alone.
- Visiting hours are determined by the hospital or the unit.
- A hospital gown may replace the patient's clothes and items such as watch, glasses, wallet, money, false teeth, and jewelry may need to be relinquished.
- A multitude of questions are asked numerous times, some of them extremely personal; feedback on the significance of the information is rarely provided.

- Physical examinations are conducted by numerous professionals, often until the patient is sore, particularly when there is difficulty in determining a diagnosis.
- Behaviors that are considered normal at home are considered out of place in the hospital. For example, if a husband gets into bed with his wife and is holding her, this can become a topic of conversation among the health care professionals.
- In addition to the invasion of the patient's privacy and space, there is most often invasion of the body.
- The patient is depersonalized when referred to as "the patient in room 216" or as "the bleeder just admitted."
- Different types of procedures and treatments are scheduled and performed, with little or no input from the patient.
- The patient may be unable to bathe without assistance.

The routines and rituals performed in the health care system are done for specific, valid reasons. This controlled environment provides an efficient and safe workplace for the nurse. Features of this setting include:

- The nurse is in one location so once at work no more travel is involved.
- The physical environment is safe and, if situations or conflicts arise, a security staff is usually available to respond.
- Coworkers in the immediate vicinity are available for collaboration when questions about nursing practice are raised, and a second opinion is welcomed.
- A variety of departments are on-site with services that can be accessed by telephone, for example, pharmacy and dietary.
- Interdisciplinary team is readily available and accessible for referrals or consultation.
- Hospital routines facilitate order and predictability of accomplishing medical and nursing goals.
- Schedules establish an orderly sequence of events.
- The equipment and supplies that are needed for patient care are just a few steps away or can be ordered from another department by telephone. Replacement and maintenance of equipment is carried out on an orderly and systematic basis.
- Although the nurse is probably exposed to more organisms in the hospital than in other settings, universal/standard precautions are strictly enforced and the nurse has access to information about specific types of infection that may be involved. Isolation equipment and supplies are readily available in the hospital setting.
- The patient is expected to be compliant and can be labelled noncompliant by the staff and treated accordingly. Only

▶ TABLE 1–1. CHARACTERISTICS OF THE ROLES OF THE NURSE AND PATIENT IN THE HOSPITAL SETTING

Nurse	Patient
Maintains control of the situation	Stripped of personal power
Practices in a safe environment	Admitted to a strange environment
Enjoys collaboration with colleagues	Experiences loneliness and dependency on the system
Works with routines and schedules	Expected to be compliant
Has support of numerous services and departments	Family/friends often not a part of medical care
Access to equipment and supplies	
Able to document on site	
Only obtains glimpses of patient's life-style	Perceives that life-style is often not taken into consideration

glimpses of life-style may be evident and the care proceeds regardless of the patient's life-style.

- Documentation can usually be completed within a short span of time and is done either manually or by computer. The forms and necessary equipment are readily available.
- The institution is controlled by its policies, rules and regulations.

The nurse in the hospital is supported in every way by the control that the institution exercises over patients and their treatments. Table 1–1 summarizes the experiences of the nurse and patient in the hospital setting.

Practicing Nursing in the Community

The situation is completely reversed when the patient is at home or in the community. This means that the patient, not the nurse, is in control. In fact, the patient is now often called a "client." Webster defines "client" as someone who is dependent. To be dependent does not necessarily mean to be "passive." The client may be dependent on the nurse and other personnel from the agency for medical care, nursing care, and assistance related to illness, but that may be the only area of the client's life where there is dependency. From this aspect, the specialty of community based nursing is very different from nursing in the hospital. To develop a perspective about nursing care of the client in the community, let us focus on some of these differences. Table 1–2 summarizes the characteristics of the nurse and client in the community setting.

► TABLE 1–2. CHARACTERISTICS OF THE ROLE OF THE NURSE AND CLIENT IN THE COMMUNITY SETTING

Nurse	Client
Practice in an unknown environment in which safety is a concern	Knows the environment
Experiences limited collaboration	Supports in place (family/friends/pets)
Often practices alone	
Is subjected to client's routines/schedules	Is in control of personal items, routines/schedules
Must adapt to client situation/life-style	Maintains self determination, living life-style

Client's Perspective

Home is where individuals can be themselves. The quality of home life can range from being happy and well-adjusted to being unhappy and maladjusted. Nonetheless, it is home. Many aspects of a person's life demonstrate that the client is in control within the home setting and while functioning within the community. If the nurse goes into the client's home during her work day, many aspects of the client's home life will be apparent. If the client is at a community based agency, the nurse must be aware that many aspects of the client's life impact his health even though they may not be obvious. These aspects include life-styles, available support systems, pets, transportation needs, and the general environment.

LIFE-STYLES. Life-styles are decided upon by individuals and their families whether or not they are aware of making the related decisions. Some people's lives are very orderly and predictable. At the opposite end of that spectrum are lives that are chaotic, unorganized, and crisis-driven. People choose when they get up and when they go to bed; some people are naturally "night" people and others are "day" people.

When people know that they make choices and that their decisions determine their lives, they feel that they are in control of their situations. This is referred to as internal locus of control. External locus of control occurs when people feel as if their environment, which includes other people, decide what happens to them; they perceive that they have little or no control over their lives or anything else. The nurse who gently involves the client in his care, making certain to stay within his limits, is supporting the client in the control his life.

SUPPORT SYSTEM. Some families have strong support systems in place. This support can be provided by family members from both inside and outside of the home. Extended family members may take turns traveling and caring for family members. Friends and neighbors may make themselves available for transportation, shopping, trips to the physician's office, providing meals, staying with the client, and just checking to see if everything is all right.

Other clients live alone and have no family or friends on whom to depend. They may live in isolated areas or be in the middle of a city. For whatever reason, they are truly alone with no support system.

 exercise 1–3: pets

A patient had a bird for a pet. He would talk to this creature and the bird made sounds in response. A family member let the bird out of his cage, in the other room, while the nurse was changing the dressing on the patient's large abdominal wound. The bird flew low and directly over the site several times in an attempt to get to the patient.

Make a list of what needs to be done and what needs to be discussed with the client about this situation. Prioritize the list.

1. Explain to the pt. the need for sterile conditions.
2. Request that the bird be returned to the cage until procedure completed.
3.

PETS. Pets can play a very significant role in the life of a client. A "watch dog" can make a family feel safe. Other animals provide companionship and love. Animals in some homes are well disciplined and follow orders whereas animals in other homes seem to do what is natural to them, including eliminating inside the house.

In whatever setting you are practicing, you need to consider pets when you are performing a procedure on a client. This is also true in your client teaching. If the client/care giver is performing a procedure, it is imperative that she understand the implications of a pet being near or having access to her body while her hands are occupied during a procedure. Pets can also raise serious issues in other community based settings, like a school classroom.

 exercise 1–4

A child in third grade, who put a box over a bat that his cat had caught, brought the live captured creature to school so his classmates could see it. What are the potential hazards of this innocent action? What is the school nurse's role in this situation?

1. Animal (bat) bite (disease may/may not result).
2. Animal escaping.

The role of the school nurse is to first educate student; to ensure safety of students; to educate families re: potential hazards.

TRANSPORTATION. The family may have a car and someone to assist with transportation for health related activities, such as getting prescriptions and supplies or helping the client get to a medical appointment. For other families with no transportation, this process is a struggle.

GENERAL ENVIRONMENT. The client and/or family are accustomed to how they live. There are environments that are orderly, neat, and clean and there are those that are cluttered, not clean, noisy, and lacking in basic necessities. If the nurse sees a client in a community based agency, she may be unable to determine if the client's environment enhances or detracts from changes related to health issues that she is helping the client to accomplish.

Nurse's Perspective

The nurse who is working in the community, whether at an agency or making home visits, must remind herself that the client has greater control over his life than the patient in the hospital. This is demonstrated by how he handles agency appointments and how he follows through with his care and recommended measures. The nurse may encounter different situations that require knowledge and adaptability, a caring yet firm approach. We will now consider a sampling of those issues.

TRANSPORTATION. Whenever you have a passenger in your car, you are liable. If a client and/or family member needs transportation from their home to a medical facility or from one agency to another and they ask you to take them, how would you respond? Your response can include that policy does not permit transporting anyone. This may not be easy for you to say, especially if you are on your way to the same destination. However, you do not want to make yourself unnecessarily vulnerable.

WORKING INDEPENDENTLY. Being out in the field, whether on a continuous basis or sporadically, has its advantages and disadvantages. There is some flexibility in planning your day as you prioritize your activities. You may be traveling and working alone. As a result, you may be concerned that you do not have the answer to a question. Tell the client or family member that you will obtain the information and either call them back or have the information for them on your next visit. Of course, if the information is needed immediately, call the appropriate person to get the answer. Most of the time, you will know more than the client and the family about the situation.

It is better to say that you do not know than to give inaccurate information. One of the primary disadvantages of working alone is that if you have a question about what you are looking at or what you are hearing, such as lung sounds, there is no one you can consult. If something is urgent, you can call your office, the physician's office, or even 911.

INFECTION CONTROL. The use of universal/standard precautions protects you in most situations in the community. Undiagnosed airborne diseases such as tuberculosis pose the same threat as in the hospital. It may be more difficult to follow up on your concerns about infection control in the community setting because you do not have the control that you do in the hospital. For example, in the hospital, the physician is available and accessible for questions you may have about the patient. Although this follow up process may take longer when practicing in the community, it is still important that you address your concerns about any communicable diseases.

SELF DETERMINATION.   People choose how they live their lives whether their choice is deliberate or not. We all know that people have the right to do this; however, in the hospital, this behavior is not often seen in action. In the community setting, a client's desire to maintain control of his life may dominate, even when continued actions go against what is best for his health. The situations and conditions you encounter in the community may be based on beliefs that are contrary to yours and may raise strong issues and feelings within you that you will need to address. For instance, you may not agree with the client who understands the rationales for life supporting changes but does not follow through on any suggestions or recommendations. This is a demonstration of the right to self determination. Sometimes, acceptance and appreciation of the client are all that we have to offer.

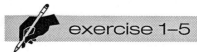

exercise 1–5

What are your feelings about clients who do not follow the prescribed medical regime?

That we as health care providers need to assess the client and the need for the regime and come up with alternatives more suitable to the client. Also need to assess barriers and how they might be overcome. If still not followed, accept autonomy of client.

Public Health Nursing and Community Health Nursing

The features that distinguish community health nursing from public health nursing are interesting. These terms are used in much the same way we use the words health and illness. We often use them synonymously. For example, we talk about a health care system that offers sick care and we have health insurance that we use when we are sick. Health and sickness are used as if the meanings of the words were the same.

Community health nursing and public health nursing are often referred to in a similar way. One receives a graduate degree from a school of public health to be able to teach community health nursing in a baccalaureate nursing program. The theory course, clinical course, and textbook are entitled community health nursing. All of this qualifies the graduate to become a public health nurse.

To clarify the two terms, let us first discuss community health nursing. Practice areas other than public health nursing and hospital nursing were labelled as community health nursing. This classification included nursing in areas such as in physicians' offices, various kinds of clinics, and adult daycare centers. Today, this would also include community based settings such as hospice and home health. The place or the setting, rather than the specific practice within these settings, determined what was considered community health nursing. Community health nursing now has a new name: community based nursing.

Public health nursing is a specialty of nursing that synthesizes public health sciences and nursing practice. The public health sciences include subjects like biostatistics, ecology, epidemiology, and nutrition. Public health nursing is determined by practice rather than setting. The goal of this specialty is health promotion and disease prevention in populations or groups of people. Examples of various types of populations are: the elderly, school-aged children, the non-insured, workers in a plant, and pregnant teenagers.

In community based nursing, the concepts of health promotion and levels of prevention are directed mainly toward individuals and families. The type of agency determines which level of prevention or if health promotion is emphasized. For example, a client dying from cancer and her family are visited by a Hospice nurse; a home care nurse visits an 85 year old man with cardiac problems living alone for blood work, assessments, and teaching; a homeless person with multiple chronic illnesses is seen at the clinic for the uninsured and undersured; and a mother brings her young infant who has diarrhea into the rural medical center. Figure 1–1 illustrates the difference in focus between public health and community based nursing.

Health Promotion

Health promotion is the effort to maintain and improve an already healthy state. In promotion of health, a problem does not exist. Mea-

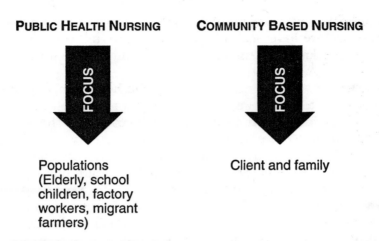

PUBLIC HEALTH NURSING

FOCUS

Populations
(Elderly, school
children, factory
workers, migrant
farmers)

COMMUNITY BASED NURSING

FOCUS

Client and family

Figure 1–1. Foci of public health nursing and community based nursing.

sures to promote health are focused on enhancing an already healthy state of being. It is important to remember that clients who are very ill may still have aspects of healthy functioning in their lives.

Prevention consists of measures that protect one from disease. It is the effort one makes to protect oneself or others from specific diseases and their consequences. There are three levels of prevention: primary, secondary, and tertiary. In teaching clients to take care of themselves, you will very often need to teach all three levels of prevention.

Levels of Prevention

Primary prevention measures focus on preventing a problem before it occurs. Strategies include immunizations, safety measures such as wearing seat belts, and health education. A good way to identify this level of prevention is to put it to a test: **one never knows if what one did was effective.** For example, many people who are not immunized never contract specific diseases and other people who do not wear seat belts are unharmed in accidents. (This is only a method of identifying the level of prevention, not a case against the measures!) The focus of both promotion of health and primary prevention is to increase health and prevent illness. It is difficult to measure the success of these strategies.

Secondary prevention consists of measures that focus on early diagnosis and prompt treatment. The entire range of screening tests (x rays, lab tests, etc.) are in this category. Examples of these tests are mammograms, Pap smears, and blood pressure measurements. The intent of this level of prevention is to identify individuals who have early symptoms of disease so they may be treated as soon as possible. If the condition cannot be cured, hopefully further complications and disability will be minimal.

Tertiary prevention activities focus on rehabilitation of a person with a disease. An example is an amputee learning to use and care for his prosthesis. An important point to remember about this level of prevention is that the person is already experiencing an acute or chronic condition when these measures are implemented. Such measures are not prescribed for healthy people, like teaching a diabetic to self-administer insulin or teaching related to chemotherapy treatments. Both secondary and tertiary levels of prevention focus on decreasing the consequences of health problems that already exist.

All three levels of prevention are addressed in public health nursing with emphasis placed on primary prevention. The purpose of an initial visit by a public health nurse could be for primary prevention. When a client goes to a community based agency because of a specific condition or disease, the focus will naturally include secondary and tertiary prevention strategies. Primary prevention may or may not be stressed, depending on the agency. However, the family can benefit from primary prevention measures such as learning effective body mechanics in caring for the client and getting enough rest. Additional public health concepts will be presented in Chapter 6.

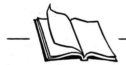

CHAPTER HIGHLIGHTS

1. The relationship of the nurse to the client in the community differs from the relationship of the nurse to the patient in the hospital.

2. Community based nursing practice includes client control in health related issues.

3. Public health nursing is population focused.

4. Community based nursing is client and family focused.

5. Promotion of health and primary prevention are directed at maintaining health or wellness.

6. Secondary and tertiary prevention are determined by client needs that relate to existing health problems.

REFERENCE

McKinnon, T.H. (1997). *Community Health Nursing: A Case Study Approach.* New York: Lippincott-Raven p. 42.

2.

Overview of the Health Care System

To understand the extent of the changes taking place in the health care system and their effect on community based nursing, we will focus on paradigms, paradigm shifts, and some of the major past events and present trends that support these changes. This knowledge will help to maintain a healthy perspective about the current state of health care in this country.

PARADIGMS AND A PARADIGM SHIFT

In his video, "The Business of Paradigms," Joel Barker states that a **paradigm is the way we think about things** (Barker, 1989). We have paradigms or <u>sets of rules and regulations about everything in our lives</u>. Some of the characteristics of paradigms are: (1) they establish a set of rules; (2) they create boundaries; and (3) they act as filters for new information.

It is helpful to apply the above concepts to a particular paradigm in the health care system. A traditional paradigm in nursing was that nursing care was separate from the cost of that care. The set of rules of that paradigm included the belief that no matter what the patient needed, the cost was unimportant to the nurse and the nurse's documentation of the care given was unrelated to reimbursement.

In following this paradigm, nurses knew the boundaries that related to the care of patients and the elements that constituted acceptable practice, such as going to another floor to borrow what was needed. These boundaries provided the framework within which quality care was safely and effectively administered. Success was based on nursing care in and of itself with no connection to the cost of that care. The nurse was valued and could easily find a job.

Another aspect of any paradigm is that it acts as a filter through which new information is viewed. If the information does not fit, the paradigm is automatically skipped over. It is not even seen or heard so it is not surprising that the message in the new information is disregarded. Nurses once believed that nothing would interfere with the care of their patients, not even concerns from administration about cutting costs. Caring and costs were not connected.

Knowledge about the origins and implications of paradigms can be very valuable, especially when a paradigm shift occurs. A **paradigm shift** is a new paradigm that is in the process of replacing the old. When this occurs, the old set of rules and boundaries no longer apply. Even the people who are working with the new paradigm have no rules or boundaries, so "everyone goes back to zero." Successful functioning in the old paradigm does not guarantee success in the new paradigm.

A major paradigm shift, cutting health care costs, has taken place within the health care system. This has created major changes, or paradigm shifts, in virtually every institution and agency in our health care system. In nursing, the shift has been from caring for patients without being involved in cost containment to being directly involved in considering the cost of that care.

The new paradigm of reducing health care costs is creating major financial constraints in institutions, leading to downsizing. Nothing seems to work as it did before and everyone is scrambling around not knowing what to do or how to deal with the new changes.

Eventually, the new paradigm will be in place. Until then, departments and services within health care facilities and agencies are undergoing reorganization, a process that is resulting in the elimination of nursing positions. In many hospitals, nursing positions are scarce and job security is rapidly diminishing. The 1995 Third Report of the PEW Health Professions Commission predicts that managed care will cause the closure of many hospitals. This trend will, in turn, affect the jobs of 350,000 nurses in these institutions who will then be seeking employment in nonhospital settings (The Home Care Marketer, 1996). The following section is a brief history of the developments that led to this paradigm shift.

HISTORICAL PERSPECTIVE

Sick people have been taken care of by their family members and others in the home throughout history. Before the mid 1800s, when mass printing began, much of what is written as history is subject to speculation and interpretation. However, it is known that people in general were poorly educated, impoverished, and forced to live in unsanitary conditions. There were continuous epidemics and the exact causes of them were unknown because the germ theory had not yet been developed. There were very few hospitals and they were places where the poor went to die. Insane asylums isolated the mentally ill from society. Professional nursing, health departments, and community agencies as we know them today did not exist. The following are some of the events that eventually contributed to the development of community based nursing.

The Epidemiological Society of London, in 1854–1856, wanted to teach poor women how to care for the sick poor in their homes. William Rathbone, whose terminally ill wife was given excellent nursing care by a nurse at home, recommended to the community authorities in 1856 that 18 districts be created and that one nurse be assigned to care for the sick in each district. In this way, the nursing needs of the community could be met. This concept was so well accepted that voluntary agencies implemented the above model on a national level in England.

Evolution of Public Health Nursing, Home Nursing, and Community Based Nursing in the United States

In 1877, the first organization to employ a graduate nurse to provide nursing care to the sick at home was the Women's Branch of the New York City Mission. Only lay persons had previously provided home nursing services.

Similar services were provided by another voluntary agency in Buffalo, New York, in 1885 and then by others in Boston and Philadelphia in 1886. A voluntary or non-official agency is one supported by donations and contributions made by citizens. These agencies later became the Visiting Nurse Associations (VNAs) (Rice, 1996). The VNAs provided nursing care to the sick in the home and became the foundation for home health nursing.

Lillian Wald established a district nursing service in the Lower East Side of New York City in 1893, called the House on Henry Street.

The dispensary was very similar to our advanced practice nurse centers of today because it was nurse-operated and controlled. The immigrants lived in crowded conditions, and poverty and sickness were common. She focused on the health needs of that population, specifically addressing those needs through communicable disease nursing, school nursing, tuberculosis nursing, and maternal–child nursing. Lillian Wald was the pioneer of public health nursing in this country. Much of the nursing care provided was home care nursing. The House on Henry Street later became the VNA of New York City (Swanson & Albrecht, 1993). By 1890, there were 21 VNAs in the United States.

Wald explained the positive impact home nursing was having on individuals and families to an official of the Metropolitan Life Insurance Company. Starting in 1909, coverage for home nursing was provided for that company's industrial policyholders (Smith & Maurer, 1995). This was an early model for the present day home care industry.

Local health departments concentrated their efforts on communicable disease control and sanitation issues. The first nurses were hired by health departments around 1900. The public health nurse focused on populations, individuals, and families. She did home care nursing, too. This service was considered a community service.

The nursing care given by both the VNAs and the local health departments over the years was of high quality and low cost. The public health nurse was able to focus on nursing practice and was not directly concerned with cost issues; state and local taxes supported the health departments and their services. The VNAs, as voluntary agencies, were supported by contributions, and there was no governmental reimbursement. Commercial health care organizations were unable to thrive. In fact, the Metropolitan Life Insurance Company's involvement in home care ceased in 1953 due to rising costs.

The development and advancement of medical technology and scientific medicine that occurred after World War II precipitated major changes in hospitals. Before these developments, hospitals were places where the poor went for treatment and, often, to die. They could not afford to pay for a physician to make home visits or for someone to perform nursing duties in the home. Those who could pay did not go to hospitals but were treated by a physician at his or her office or at home.

World War II was the impetus that created a shift from physicians treating patients in their offices and in the patient's home to the hospital. Hospital construction was subsidized through the passage of the

Hill–Burton Act of 1946 which led to a proliferation of hospitals. These determining factors moved the hospital from a welfare institution to a complex industry.

As physicians treated more patients in the hospital and visited fewer patients in their homes, nurses from the VNAs and the health department made more home visits. For-profit home health agencies were rare. This was to change with the passage of the Medicare and Medicaid programs by Congress in 1965.

Governmental Involvement in Health Care

The purpose of Medicare is to ensure medical care for the aged and disabled, which includes substituting home care for hospitalization and extended care. Medicare Part A covers hospital costs, and Part B covers medical charges. The program is federally funded by taxes applied to wages and premiums paid by those receiving the benefits (entitled beneficiaries). As the cost of medical care has risen, so has the cost of implementing the Medicare program. In 1967, the Medicare budget was $4.7 billion compared to $194 billion in 1996. (Anders, 1997).

Medicaid was passed by Congress along with Medicare. Medicaid is a grant program administered by each state. Its purpose is to provide medical assistance to people below certain income levels. The federal government pays each state according to its need and the states finance the remaining amount with general tax revenues. The federal government supports Medicaid through taxes levied against income. Medicaid provides health care for more than 28 million people or one in ten Americans (Weiss, 1997).

The implementation of Medicare and Medicaid programs put the government into the business of health care. Now there was a source of income for health care providers and the number of home care agencies in this country increased from 1100 in 1963 to more than 17,500 in 1995 (National Association for Home Care, 1995). In addition to the increased numbers of agencies, there was a marked change in the direction of home care.

Before the passage of these programs, home care was managed by nurses. Physicians directed only the medical aspects of patient care such as orders for procedures and medications. The government's investment in health care naturally led to the monitoring of who could receive the services of the programs. Physicians were awarded the role of gatekeeper by the government, thereby shifting the management of home care from nursing to medicine. A direct consequence is that nursing is responsible for the home care of patients (approximately 90% of home health agency visits today are nursing visits) but nursing is no longer in control. This accounts for the emphasis on a client population that has medical problems and treatments for which reimbursement is available. Health promotion and primary prevention are usually not reimbursed.

 exercise 2-1

Try to put yourself in the place of the physician for a moment. You think that certain diagnostic tests should be performed on a patient to rule out certain conditions or diseases. The insurance company states it will not pay for the tests you think are necessary. In the past, you were the one who decided what was ordered and insurance coverage was not a question. Now limitations are put on the way you practice.

How do you feel about this paradigm shift?

....

....

....

....

....

....

List the pros and cons of this situation.

....

....

....

....

....

....

MANAGED CARE

We need to pause a moment to examine the concept of managed care and identify various associated terms and structures. **Managed care** relates to the management of patient care and therefore has been in existence since there have been patients. The present day concept of managed care emerged in the 1980s in an attempt to reduce health care costs. Ideally, managed care is quality health care delivered in a cost-effective way, with prudent monitoring of access to resources. Very basically, it relates to any health system that has an entity other than the patient or the health care giver, such as an insurance company, that influences the kind of care delivered to the patient. This entity can intervene and decide the care that is appropriate for the patient (Cohen & Cesta, 1997). Unfortunately, managed care is money driven, which is evidenced by new expressions such as "cost-per-life."

FINANCING OF HEALTH CARE

Payment for health care in our country is about evenly divided between private and public sources. Private sources are voluntary, charitable, and all monies other than from a governmental source. Public or governmental sources are tax generated. Figure 2–1 illustrates the breakdown of health care payments by private and public sources.

Types of Reimbursement Structures

There are various types of reimbursement methods and models through which health care is financed, as discussed below.

Fee-for-Service
Payment occurs after the service is provided. An example is the patient who sees his physician and is then billed at a later date.

Prospective Payment
Payment is made to the provider in advance of service and is based on a prediction of cost.

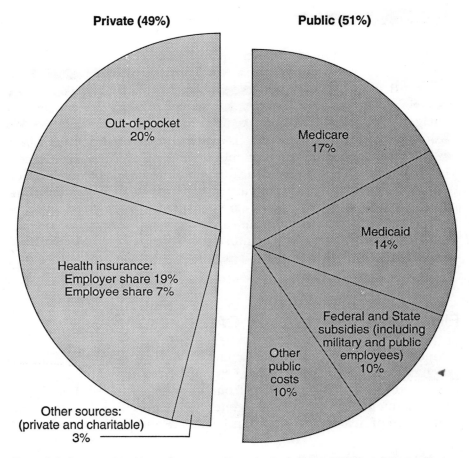

Figure 2–1. Sources of health care payments. *(From the Department of Health and Human Services, 1992).*

Co-payment

Payment is a fixed amount no matter how much a service costs. Some-times, co-payment is referred to as the allotted part of the bill for which the patient is responsible for paying. The insurance company or other organization pays a specified amount and the patient pays the difference between this amount and the total amount charged. For ex-ample, if a medical service is $50.00 and the insurance company pays $35.00, the patient pays the co-payment of $15.00.

Third-party Payment

Payment is made by a third party or the intermediary between the physician and the patient, such as an insurance company. The third party is billed by the physician and the physician is paid directly by this organization. The patient is not involved in the payment to the physician. This process of payment is believed to cause people to use their insurance more than if they are directly involved in the payment. An analogy is the use of credit cards versus the use of cash. A person will usually spend less when using cash than when using a credit card.

Capitation

A payment system whereby one fixed fee, monthly or annually, is paid to a health care provider to cover all services provided.

The cost of health care has risen dramatically since the inception of Medicare and Medicaid in 1965. These programs resulted in the government paying for the health care costs of the aged, disabled, and economically disadvantaged. Because the government ordinarily pays less than the "usual and customary" amount for services, and the economically disadvantaged are unable to pay co-payments, the providers are receiving less for their services to these beneficiaries. In order to make up some of the difference between what was paid and what was expected to be paid, the providers have increased the cost of service to patients who are able to pay. This practice is known as **cost-shifting**. In addition to this phenomenon, costly technological advances, unnecessary medical procedures, inflation, and third-party payment have also contributed to massive increases in health care costs.

Types of Managed Care Organizations

Pre-paid health plans were viewed as a potential way of decreasing health care costs in the 1960s. The label **health maintainance organization** (HMO) emerged in the 1970s, and the number of HMOs grew. Today, there are many types of HMOs that have the goal of providing comprehensive health care on a pre-paid basis to an enrolled group. The patient is charged a monthly rate whether or not services are used and there may be co-payments attached to specific services. The HMO either provides for or agrees to pay for stipulated services. The focus is on preventive care. HMOs are involved with physicians in a variety of ways.

- *Staff model*: physicians employed directly by the HMO
- *Group practice model*: a contract with groups of multi-specialty physicans

- *Network model:* a contract with a network of physicians to cover the range of needs of participants.
- *Independent practice association (IPA) model:* an association of individual physicians who offer services to participants (Cohen and Cesta, 1997)

Exploding increases in health care costs led to the passage of the 1983 Amendments to the Social Security Act (Public Law 98-21.) This legislation resulted in the establishment of **Diagnostic Related Groups** (DRGs), a payment system for hospital care that is linked to a specific number of days per medical diagnosis. For example, if a diagnosis requires three hospital days and the patient is discharged in two, the hospital keeps the money for the third hospital day. Obviously, it is to the hospital's advantage to discharge a patient as soon as possible. DRGs were the catalyst for early discharge of sicker patients, the recent explosive growth in home care agencies, and the increased numbers of nurses practicing home care nursing.

Although the purpose of DRGs was to contain costs, this process caused more cost-shifting onto the insurance companies who, in turn, passed the cost to businesses providing health insurance to their employees. Businesses then increased employee insurance premiums or held wages down to cover costs.

Businesses pay approximately 20% of the nation's health care costs and they were outraged at the increased costs of health insurance premiums. Insurance companies and other companies began putting together HMOs and other cost-effective programs. The growth of these health plans is seen in the number of hospitals participating in HMOs which has increased from 48% in 1986 to 98% in 1996 (Cohen and Cesta, 1997).

Another type of managed care organization developed as health care providers began to contract with various businesses and insurance companies to give discounts for services to their employees. These managed care organization are known as **preferred provider organizations** (PPOs). The cost of care to the employee is less for services from a PPO. An example is an office visit that costs $50.00: The cost to an employee for using the physician on the PPO list may be $5.00 compared to $18.00 for a physician not on the list.

A third type of managed care organization is the **point-of-service** (POS) **plan.** In this plan, the primary care physician is the gatekeeper for hospital admissions, specialists, emergency, and other services. There is a fixed fee for services. If the patient chooses to receive services outside of this provider network, the patient must pay the cost.

Case Management

Managed care provides the overall structure for cost-effective care. Within that structure you will find nursing case management. **Case management** is a process for planning, coordinating, and monitoring patient care across health care settings. This processs extends from treatment to recovery, securing needed services and resources while promoting health and containing costs. The case manager usually coordinates nursing care rather than providing the direct patient care.

The use of a critical path or pathways ensures that the patient receives needed care on a timely basis. **Critical pathways** are based on predetermined criteria and a plan for the day to day expectations for a patient with a specific diagnosis. Multidisciplinary action plans are called MAPS. The use of MAPS makes it possible for each discipline to track the patient's progress on a daily basis.

In addition to development of these structures and mechanisms, there are societal trends that are having an impact on community based nursing.

TRENDS INFLUENCING NURSING CARE

Many forces have contributed to the rapid development of community based nursing. Among them are advanced technology, increased mobility of family members, changes within the family, and the growth of the aging population.

Technology

The practice of early discharge of very ill patients from the hospital who need specialized care has increased the demand for services that many community based agencies can provide. The care of these less stable, more acutely ill people in the community requires advanced technology and the need for staff nurses with the expertise to work with this equipment. This trend has also placed a greater burden on family members and non-professional caregivers to monitor this technology.

Increased Mobility of Family Members

Our society is very mobile. The nuclear family and extended family are no longer in close proximity; members often live hundreds, if not thousands, of miles away from each other. When a family member needs assistance for a period of time, it is very possible that no one in the family will be available to provide the necessary care.

Changes Within the Family

There are increasing numbers of single-parent families within the United States population. Many females are now heads of households. This trend can have serious implications for the support system of the family. Traditionally, women have been the nurturers of their families. However, more and more women are employed outside the home, whether single or married; as a result, they are just not as available to care for sick or aged family members. This is especially true for family members who are experiencing chronic conditions or illnesses. As families relinquish their responsibilities for the care of members, there is little or no role modeling for younger members. This raises the question: If family members did not participate in the caregiving of any of its members, at some later date even if they were able, would they feel comfortable in that role?

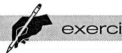 exercise 2-2

What do you think it takes to be a caregiver over time? What is involved? Make a list.

....

....

....

....

....

....

....

....

....

....

Aging Population

Another trend that is having a significant impact on health care is the extended lifespan. Today, life expectancy is 79 years for women and 72 years for men. The frail elderly—those 80 years old and older—are increasing in numbers. The needs of this group require a large percentage of the available health care resources. As a culture, we place people above a certain age in a category identified as either aged, older adult, or elderly and eliminate descriptive terms such as parent or grandparent. In contrast, we do not often refer to children as "the young." Is it possible that this depersonalization of an entire segment of our population makes it easier for society in general to tolerate the way aged parents and grandparents are treated?

 exercise 2–3

Close your eyes and think of the term "aged population." Now think of the term "aged parents." Is there a different feeling to each term? Describe your feelings associated with each term.

....

....

....

....

....

....

Although the new paradigm is causing continuous change, it presents opportunities for innovative thinking and creative nursing practice. It is important to remember that our health care system is not synchronized; it is fragmented. This means that some agencies use case managers; others do not. Some community based agencies rely heavily on public funds; others depend on private monies. Study the community agency you are involved with and share this information with your peers. This sharing will help you to grasp the mosaic of available nursing care.

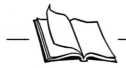

CHAPTER HIGHLIGHTS

1. The health care system in the United States is experiencing a paradigm shift.

2. The government has become a dominant force in health care.

3. Managed care is a response to the explosive growth in health care costs.

4. The mechanisms of managed care represent ways of distributing resources for health care.

5. Several major trends, such as advanced technology, increased mobility of families, changes within the family structure and the aging population, support the expansion of community based nursing.

REFERENCES

Anders, G. Estimate of improper Medicare costs soars. *The Wall Street Journal,* June 11, 1997.

Barker, J. (1989). The Business of paradigms. (Video.) *Discovering the Future Series.* Burnsville, MN: CHARTHOUSE International (800-328-3789).

Cohen, E. & Cesta, T. (1997) *Nursing Case Management.* (2nd ed.) St. Louis: Mosby.

The Home Care Marketer. (1996). *Ideas for Home Care Providers.* September/ October.

National Association for Home Care. (1995). *Basic Statistics About Home Care 1995.* Washington, DC.

Rice, R. (1996). *Home Health Nursing Practice: Concepts and Application.* (2nd ed.) St. Louis: Mosby.

Smith, C. & Maurer, F. (1995). *Community Health Nursing.* Philadelphia: Saunders.

Swanson, J. & Albrecht, M. (1993). *Community Health Nursing: Promoting the Health of Aggregates.* Philadelphia: Saunders.

Weiss, L. D. (1997). *Private Medicine and Public Health.* Boulder, CO: Westview Press.

II.

PERSPECTIVES OF THE NURSE

3.

Personal Perspectives
of the Nurse

This chapter focuses on you—what you believe about your role as nurse and the role of client. Your beliefs can determine the outcome of your nursing practice. Many of these beliefs are very subtle and we are often unaware of their presence. A discussion about beliefs and several experiential exercises are provided to heighten your awareness of how you view yourself, your clients, and their families.

In addition to beliefs, we will explore the issue of boundaries, taking care of yourself and others, and various personal skills. The characteristics of a community based nurse and the relationship between the nurse and the client, in that role, are discussed.

THE IMPACT OF BELIEFS

Each one of us has beliefs about everything and those beliefs determine how we live and what we experience (Palmer, 1994). For example, if a high school student does not believe she can attend college, what do you think her chances are of going? She may say, "I can't afford it" (a belief), or "I'm not smart enough" (a belief), or "my father said I can't" (a belief).

Another high school student, one who is planning to attend college, may say, "I want to be a nurse" (a belief) or "I plan to study nursing at a university" (a belief), or "I'll need to work while I'm going to school" (a belief). The clearer a student's beliefs are about this decision, the greater his chance of attending college and completing the requirements for a degree. The student's achievements in college will also depend on beliefs.

Now let's look at a third example, the student whose parents want him to attend college (a belief), but he does not really want to go (a belief). He believes that he ought to go to college because his parents expect it of him. His parents send for the application, but he procrastinates when it comes to filling it out and never quite gets around to completing what is required. His actions reveal what he really believes, even though he may not be aware of his beliefs related to attending college. This is known as a **transparent belief** because he is acting through the belief without being aware of it (Palmer, 1994).

Another scenario is the student whose parents want the student to be a nurse but the student wants to be a teacher. The student does not make her wishes known because she "doesn't want to disappoint her parents" (a belief). Think for a moment about the possibilities of what may happen to this student. In the end, her approach to the situation depends on her beliefs; for example "I can get through this" or "It won't be so bad" or "I can't do this."

Paying attention to what you think (self-talk) and what you say will help bring some of your beliefs to your awareness. As you begin to study community based nursing you may find yourself saying, "I really like hospital nursing. I don't want to work in the community," or "I'll keep an open mind." How will these beliefs impact your experience? Your set of beliefs about yourself or your paradigm determine your reality. The beliefs you hold have led to the professional experiences you are having today, just as the beliefs the clients hold shape their lives. The ability to recognize the connection between beliefs and reality in ourselves, and then to recognize the same relationship of beliefs to reality in clients, can provide an added dimension to nursing practice that can be valuable.

Personal Boundaries

Everyone has personal boundaries. Figuratively, this is the point where one person ends and another begins. We have many boundaries that are related to our bodies, relationships with family and friends, and material items such as property. An example of one type of boundary is a person's desk in an office environment. If another person is discovered rummaging through one's desk looking for something, without the owner's permission, the response to this situation will vary depending on the clarity of the boundaries involved and the beliefs

exercise 3–1

Briefly complete the following statements:

1. I became a nurse because . . . .

I want to give back to the community the kindness & empathy I received from nurses in the past ; to have an impact on society.

2. I made it through school because of (or in spite of) . . .

my hardwork and determination regardless of social and financial barriers.

3. and this is how I feel about it. . . .

great! I can't believe I've gotten this far. I would like to continue my education when my BSN is completed.

Now, find a partner and exchange comments. Read what your partner has written and identify the various beliefs.

Beliefs:

1. ....
2. ....
3. ....
4. ....
5. ....

Read your beliefs as recorded by your partner. Were you aware of these beliefs? Are any particular beliefs surprising or upsetting?

....

....

....

....

....

exercise 3–2

One student provides details about the exercise in which the motivation for attending nursing school is considered but not written down. The other student listens for the expression of beliefs and records them.

Beliefs:

1. ....

2. ....

3. ....

4. ....

5. ....

After recording the beliefs, the student who is recording should ask: "What were you thinking as you were doing this exercise (for example, "This is easy" or "I can't do this," and so on).

surrounding them. One person may not be bothered at all by this action, while another is outraged.

The client who is experiencing health-related problems or conditions is vulnerable and may permit the nurse (because of his beliefs about the role of nurse) to step onto his side of several boundaries where he usually permits few people or no one. As a result, the boundaries can become fuzzy or blurred between the nurse and the client. Nurses need to acknowledge that they can impinge on a client's boundaries and that this occurrence must be accompanied by a healthy respect for being in that space. For example, a client who was independent until recently and is accustomed to managing his life may be offended or pleased (depending on his beliefs surrounding that particular boundary) if the nurse takes the initiative of making an appointment for the client. Checking with the client before taking an action or making an assumption can prevent an inadvertent violation of a client's boundary.

The nurse who moves into the client's boundary but does not permit the client into many of her personal boundaries may find it easier to remain objective about the client's care. This approach helps the nurse in developing compassion and empathy for the client, but also promotes the emotional detachment between them.

 exercise 3–3

Identify a boundary you have and recall an experience when someone violated that boundary.

....

....

....

....

....

What was your reaction?

....

....

....

....

....

Did you feel it in your body?

....

....

Where?

....

....

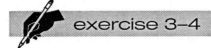

Can you recall treating a stranger differently because the person reminded you of someone close to you like your grandmother or your favorite uncle? How did your approach to this person differ from that normally taken with unfamiliar people?

....

....

....

....

....

....

The nurse who permits the client to cross her boundaries or who is not aware of her boundaries can find herself emotionally blended with the client. In this position, the nurse is as vulnerable as the client. There are advantages and disadvantages to being in this position. One of the benefits of this experience is that it can provide the nurse with the opportunity of fully learning about herself and the client. A disadvantage of this behavior is that it can result in extreme pain and emotional exhaustion caused by the attachment (opposite of detachment).

If you are unaware of your personal boundaries, you are open to anyone crossing those lines at any time. You will receive clues that this situation has occurred, after it has happened, by how you feel. Usually what one feels is an emotion, such as anger. Your body will give you clues so pay attention to the location in which you feel the emotion. Then work at identifying that emotion and respond appropriately to it.

The more you know about your boundaries, the more aware you are of what is happening while it is happening. You are then free to make a conscious choice as to who you let into specific boundaries. Once you are aware, the choice is yours.

There will be times in your career that you find yourself becoming emotionally attached to a client. You need to recognize what is happening and then decide how you are going to manage the situation. If you choose to emotionally withdraw, you need to be as gentle as possible so the client is able to make a smooth adjustment.

Aspects of Caring

There is an expression that "You teach best what you most need to learn" (Bach, 1977). There are important ideas in this statement. The first is that you can never teach another anything. You can make your skills, your knowledge, and your expertise available to another in an understandable form, but what the other person does with this information is entirely up to him or her. The second idea in this expression is that you do what you do in order to teach yourself something. In other words, whatever you are about contains what you have yet to learn.

Nurses take care of other people. Therefore, the lesson they need to learn is that they must take care of themselves! Every time we take care of someone, we are really teaching ourselves how to care for ourselves. Awareness of this concept can help you to step back and observe your nursing practice. You can accelerate the process of learning about your needs by asking questions about yourself.

In your community based nursing practice, you may see nurses who do not treat themselves well, behavior that can be manifested by such activities as avoiding the drinking of adequate amounts of fluids during the day so as to prevent the need to stop often to urinate, not stopping to eat when hungry in order to finish earlier, or ignoring signs of exhaustion instead of taking a day off once in a while to rest.

Taking care of yourself can ensure a consistent sense of well being accompanied by a high level of energy. Paying attention to your body's signals or learning what those signals are will tell you what you need to do for yourself. Take time for yourself. When you feel you have no time, that is when you especially need to have time for you. Table 3–1 poses questions for you to consider in assessing your own self-care activities.

▶ TABLE 3–1. ASSESSMENT OF SELF-CARE ACTIVITIES

Do you:
get the amount of sleep you need? Mostly
eat the diet that is best for you? Mostly
drink adequate amounts of water? No.
have enough fun and laughter in your life? Mostly
get enough affection and hugs? Yes.
have time for friendships? Yes.
commune with nature on a regular basis? No.
find time to be alone? Yes.
appreciate yourself and others? Yes.
take time to plan for what you need? Sometimes

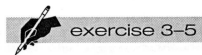

exercise 3-5

Identify areas in your life in which you would like to take better care of yourself. Imagine yourself taking care of these areas the way you would like.

More excercise, rest and water. More time for friendships.

What does this include?

Make a list of your beliefs related to taking care of yourself.

Examine the actions you take. Could you have some transparent beliefs related to taking care of yourself?

SKILLS FOR USE IN COMMUNITY BASED PRACTICE

There are many personal skills you will use in community based nursing. Everyone has them to varying degrees. You know the skills you are comfortable with and those that need improvement. Keeping your knowledge base current is a necessity whether you are practicing in an acute care setting or in a community setting. The development of your communication skills is also an on-going process.

Communication Skills

In other nursing courses, you learned communication skills and now apply them in your practice. You will be refining and expanding those skills as you practice in the community setting.

Listening skills are particularly important. Nurses need to listen intently to clients, families and/or significant others so as to hear the beliefs that support the expressed feelings, intentions, motivations, problems, and behaviors. Occasionally, it is the information that is not directly requested that can be most helpful in your nursing practice. For example, a client may discuss a concern with you that is not a direct response to a question but is pertinent to the outcome.

Verbal communication involves the use of words. The words you choose to use, the speed at which you use them, and the combination of the words you choose can make the difference of whether or not your message is understood. Listening to the level of the words that the client uses will make you aware of the kinds of words you want to use so that the client will absorb what you say.

In addition to the spoken words, you want to observe **non-verbal communication**. People may be unaware that through the use of body language, posture, the amount of space between people as they converse, body movement, gestures, and touch, they amplify the meaning of what they are saying. Are the words and the body language congruent? Are the client's arms folded across her body, indicating a closed position, as her words are trying to convey that she is open about a particular subject? The body often speaks louder than the words.

Most of what we continuously communicate about ourselves is on a non-verbal level. When someone is "present" with us, we know it. If a person is physically present, yet preoccupied and not quite with us, we know that, too. This can occur especially when you are under a lot of stress. If it does happen, bring yourself back and be with the client during the visit. Remember, your client may do this to you, too.

Communicating effectively, both orally and in writing, is a goal of the nurse. The nurse is often the leader of the community based multidisciplinary team. It is essential for team members, who may have little or no contact with each other on a daily basis in the community, to communicate effectively and for the leader to coordinate services among the providers.

 exercise 3-6

Work with a partner.

One partner plays the nurse while the other plays the client. (One student plays a client in a clinic setting and the other a client in her home.)

The student playing the nurse is talking with the client, attempting to assess his situation.

The student playing the client is physically present but obviously preoccupied.

Then switch roles.

How did you know the client was not present?

....

....

....

....

....

How did you bring the client back to the conversation?

....

....

....

....

....

Interviewing Skills

Your interaction with clients is purposeful. The use of effective interviewing skills assists the nurse in obtaining the information needed from the client and caregivers without making them feel interrogated. There are both informal and formal interviews.

The **informal interview** has the purpose of obtaining a limited amount of information. There is not a series of formalized questions so the gathering of this information can be accomplished through normal conversation. It is essential that you know which data are needed prior to the beginning of the interview. The phrasing of general statements or questions has a definite effect on the responses obtained. In just a few moments of listening to someone, you will know how to phrase and rephrase questions. A goal of the health professional during the interview is to obtain the information that is necessary for assessment, planning, and delivery of care. Very often, nonpertinent information is automatically screened out. Due to time constraints, it is often necessary for the nurse to gently direct the client to give the needed information.

The **formal interview** usually consists of a series of written questions that need to be answered for the purpose of gathering specific information. An initial work-up of a client tends to contain formalized questions whether the client is seen in a clinic, at a plant, at school, or in the home. With skill, the nurse who is very familiar with the content of the questions is able to shift back and forth from the conversation mode to asking specific questions. Some large community agencies, such as home care agencies, have nurses who conduct only initial visits. Medicare's Outcome and Assessment Information Set (OASIS-B), which is most likely to be required for each initial visit of a client who is covered by Medicare, is comprised of 79 formalized questions to be completed on the first visit (Federal Register, 1997). The purpose of this questionnaire is to measure client outcomes in home health.

CHARACTERISTICS OF THE COMMUNITY BASED NURSE

To effectively practice community based nursing, the nurse must have strengths in specific areas. These include the ability to work independently, strong critical thinking skills, organizational ability, flexibility, acceptance, and appreciation.

Working Independently

Many nurses enjoy working by themselves. They do not particularly miss the camaraderie of nurses working together and find that conferring with staff at the office is enough. There may be a trade-off between working independently and the availability of interaction of other staff. These nurses are very often inner-directed or self starters. They do not need outside stimulation or rules and regulations (other-directed) for them to get their work done. When working alone, it is important for you to know when you need to interact with others besides clients and what it takes to meet those needs.

Critical Thinking Skills

The ability to make sound decisions and use good judgment is high on the list of needed characteristics. Your assessment and evaluation skills greatly affect the identification of outcomes and planning nursing interventions. Of course, there are times when you will question your decisions, but your ability to think critically comes to the forefront. Nurses who enjoy working solo are usually secure in themselves and derive pleasure from setting priorities and making independent decisions. They know when to ask for assistance and when to proceed unassisted.

Organizational Skills

In community based settings like home care, hospice, school health, and occupational health, the nurse uses organizational skills in many activities such as planning her daily visits, selecting the necessary equipment and supplies, and ensuring that a variety of forms are available for use. These skills are blended with the application of the nursing process to each client, student, or employee. Organizational skills are also needed to balance the care of these clients and to keep abreast of the rules and regulations of both the agency, school, or company for which the nurse is employed and those of the state and federal government.

Flexibility

Community based nurses, in many settings, create most of the structure of their work and need to be flexibile in planning their days, weeks, and months. They take pleasure in determining their schedules and meeting their goals on a continuous basis. Those who need fixed routines and directives, like those found in most acute care settings, would feel very insecure functioning in the community.

Acceptance and Appreciation

Another characteristic needed by community based nurses is the acceptance of people as they are. Each person is different. It is very helpful if nurses are able to appreciate people as they find them; living their lives on their own terms. It can be a challenge at times to do the best you can do and then relinquish any investment in how the client handles his situation. In the acute care setting, the nurse is distanced from much of the patient's life.

RELATIONSHIP BETWEEN THE NURSE AND THE CLIENT/FAMILY

The success of the nurse–client relationship in community based nursing is particularly important because the client may not interact with many other professionals. If a need arises, it is important for the client to be able to express it. The professional relationship between the community based nurse and the client is enhanced by recognizing the beliefs of the client and understanding life-style differences.

Beliefs of the Client

When two people, like the client and the nurse, have similar beliefs about a particular situation or condition, there is easy agreement. For example, the nurse may believe that one follows the directions of an "expert" when it is in one's best interest. Similarly, the client believes that he will do whatever the medical experts tell him to do in order to feel better. Therefore, there is a high likelihood that whatever suggestions the nurse makes or instructions she gives, the client will follow through if at all possible.

If the beliefs of the client and those of the nurse directly oppose each other, then the nurse is presented with a challenge. If the client does not follow specific instructions even though they are in his best interest, the nurse is going to have to resolve any conflict that arises within her about this. It is acceptable, in the health care system, to use fear, threatening and punitive language, and to be impatient with clients who do not comply with the prescribed regime. If there is any hope of change within the client; it is most likely to emerge when the nurse is able to accept and appreciate where the client is. To encourage the client and reinforce any positive measures that the client is

 exercise 3–7

An initial visit is made to a 65-year-old black female who lives alone in an apartment that is located in a small town of a rural area. She is a newly-diagnosed diabetic. Her teenage neighbor is present during the home visit.

The Caucasian nurse takes her vitals, which are: BP 176/70; pulse 100; and respirations 24. Her CBG is 470. The nurse asks "What did you eat for breakfast?" She states, "A little oatmeal, toast and coffee." The next question the nurse asks is whether she "added anything" to her food. The client finally concedes she put sugar on her oatmeal and added 2–3 teaspoons of sugar to each of her three cups of coffee.

The nurse explains the seriousness of her condition to her, such as possible resulting amputations of toes, feet and legs, and what effect diabetes can have on "different body systems."

At that point, the young neighbor girl goes into the kitchen and announces, "I'm throwing this sugar away." The client responds angrily, "Leave my sugar alone!"

The nurse then tells the client that if she isn't willing to help herself, the nurse would have to stop making home visits. The nurse explains to the client that she could use substitutes like "Sweet 'n' Low" or "Equal." The client does not seem interested.

The nurse says she will be back for a follow up in a few days.

1. How would you feel if you were this client? Explain.

Angry @ being threatened.
Frustrated that I'm unable to live how I want
Ashamed for using sugar.

2. What would the nurse have to believe for the home visit to have proceeded as it did?

That she is right & the client is wrong.

3. How could the initial visit have been conducted better?

Explain the effects of sugar on diabetes.
Offer alternatives (eg Equal).
Ask if she'd be willing to supplement.
Try sugar weaning to ↓ dependence.

taking can provide hope. Sometimes people are able to change their beliefs in an instant; for example, the client who has a heart attack and never smokes again.

If the client does not comply with any suggestions, it is appropriate to compassionately tell her what you are experiencing. Ask her how she would like to proceed. She may be able to give you the information that can lead to a new approach. The client may make a suggestion as to what she needs. Being honest and authentic can save everyone time and energy.

The nurse in community based nursing is more likely to see clients over time than the nurse in the acute care setting. Health issues that are intimately linked to life-style can take time to change. The interrelatedness of the client's and the nurse's beliefs can greatly impact the progress made.

Life-Style Differences

The term "life-style" refers to how people live their lives. It is the end result, at a given moment, of a multitude of beliefs in the form of attitudes, values, emotions, judgments, hopes, dreams, expectations, and skills. These patterns of behavior can be either positive or negative. Positive patterns of behavior support wellness and include behaviors such as regular exercise and a healthy diet. Negative patterns, like smoking, have a detrimental effect on health.

Everyone has a life-style. The nurse in the acute care setting may only get an occasional glimpse of the patient's life-style because the patient is not in his environment. Nursing care of the patient proceeds with or without this information.

The community based nurse is introduced to varying amounts of the client's life-style, depending on the specific setting. The nurse who is making a home visit sees much of the client's life-style. All the nurse may need is clarification of specific details. This information is extremely valuable in planning nursing care with the client because it can provide a point of reference for how to proceed.

The employee at work, the student at school, or the client at a clinic are out of their usual environments when seen by the nurse. In spite of this, some aspects of life-style will be evident. For example, the client's grooming, clothing, and whether or not she follows through can give you some clues. Even the method of transportation can be relevant. Aspects of the client's life-style that are not apparent yet vital to your nursing care can be obtained by asking questions.

Making judgments about life-style is easy. The greater the distance or gap between your life-style and that of the client, the more it can affect the relationship. Searching for and focusing on the positive patterns or strengths is made difficult by negative judgments. For instance, your judgment about a client can be deeply influenced by the physical environment in which the client and family live. These judgments can prevent you from getting in touch with the strengths that may be present in the family, such as very strong bonds among the family members. An awareness of your beliefs and attitudes can give you the option of changing your perspective about the situation so that you will be able to focus on the client's strengths. These strengths, which you can help the client to identify, can become the force that moves the client in the direction of desired changes.

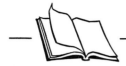

CHAPTER HIGHLIGHTS

1. Beliefs about yourself determine your reality.

2. Awareness of boundaries provides freedom of choice.

3. Nursing can provide the nurse the opportunity to learn self-care.

4. Personal skills needed in the community setting include effective communication and interview techniques.

5. Valuable characteristics for the community based nurse to possess and cultivate are: working independently, critical thinking and organizational skills, flexibility, and accepting and appreciating people.

6. Variation in the beliefs of the client and those of the nurse present challenges to the community based nurse. Assisting the client with necessary life-style changes is facilitated by a non-judgmental attitude and acceptance.

REFERENCES

Bach, R. (1997). *Illusions.* New York: Delacorte Press p. 48.
Federal Register. (1997). Vol. 62(46):11035–11064.
Palmer, H. (1994). *Resurfacing: Techniques for Exploring Consciousness.* Altamonte Springs, FL: Star's Edge International.

4.

Professional Perspectives of the Nurse

 exercise 4–1

How do you feel about the nurse who chooses not to stop to assist someone who has been in an accident or who has collapsed in a public place?

I believe it is the nurses' duty to help.

What do you think may be some of the reasons a nurse may choose not to stop?

In a hurry. Going somewhere else. Not confident of skills.

This chapter discusses concepts, issues, and information that pertain to your professional practice in general and in your safe nursing practice within any community based agency. This material includes general legal and ethical knowledge, documentation, doctor's orders, incident reports, the purpose of an agency orientation, the interdisciplinary team, community resources, and the referral process.

ETHICAL AND LEGAL ASPECTS

In this section, we will review and examine a few general concepts of ethical and legal issues that you may want to keep in mind no matter where you are, at work or in your personal life. **Ethics** is a branch of philosophy that is concerned with the rightness or wrongness of behavior. An action that is unethical may or may not be illegal. It is often difficult to know where ethics end and the law begins, or where the law ends and ethics begin. One distinguishing factor between ethics and the law is that ethics is related to conscience and the law usually

▶ TABLE 4–1. ETHICAL PRINCIPLES

Principle	Definition	Nurse's Behavior
Autonomy	Exercise of free choice	Collaborates with clients in establishing client-centered goals. Respects client's wish to refuse care.
Nonmaleficence	To do no harm	Follows medication procedure meticulously. Reports colleagues' incompetence appropriately.
Beneficence	To do good	Interacts empathically with clients. Spends time reminiscing with elderly clients.
Justice	Fair distribution of resources	Plans daily schedule to assure that the most vulnerable clients are given adequate care. Participates in professional efforts to provide health care to the homeless.
Fidelity	Faithfulness	Returns to spend time with a client after promising to do so. Supports colleague who is working to improve standards of nursing care.
Confidentiality	Protection of private, personal information	Refuses to discuss hospitalized colleague's condition with non–health-care providers. Does not obtain unnecessary information.
Veracity	Truthfulness	Reports and records accurately. Admits own errors immediately.

Reproduced, with permission, from Berger K. J. & Williams M. A. (1992). Fundamentals of Nursing: Collaborating for Optimal Health. East Norwalk, CT: Appleton & Lange.

involves some sort of material penalty (Haddad & Kapp, 1991). An-other difference between ethics and the law is that answers to ethical issues are not perfect while the answers to legal issues are either right or wrong (Guido, 1997).

The ethical principles of autonomy, nonmaleficence, benefi-cence, justice, fidelity, confidentiality, and veracity are defined and examples of applicable nursing behaviors, are given for each in Ta-ble 4–1.

There are seven types of laws: common, civil, public, criminal, pri-vate, substantive, and procedural. Tort law is a specialty of civil law. Professional nurses need to pay particular attention to this area of law (Guido, 1997). Table 4–2 lists torts and gives examples of offenses of each.

Good Samaritan Laws

Good Samaritan laws were enacted to encourage health care providers to assist strangers in emergency situations without risk of criminal and civil liability. Each state has Good Samaritan laws, and they differ

▶ TABLE 4–2. TYPES AND EXAMPLES OF TORTS

Tort / Lawsuit	Sample Description of Offense
Fraud	Misrepresentation of credentials; falsification of a client's records
Invasion of privacy	Sharing confidential information; refusing to allow use of personal clothing when it would not interfere with pro-cedures; demonstrating a procedure on a client with-out permission
Slander (defamation of character	Making a false verbal statement about a client having a socially unacceptable disease (eg, AIDS) to another health professional
Libel (defamation of character	Making a false statement about a client in writing or making such a statement to mass media (press, tele-vision)
Assault	Threatening or appearing to threaten to provide treat-ment without consent
Battery	Treating a client without consent
False imprisonment	Restraining a client inappropriately; detaining a client in a treatment facility against his or her will
Negligence	Negligence is the tort—but with licensed providers it is often called malpractice
Malpractice (negligence)	Failure to maintain expected standards of care

greatly from state to state. The following list shows you the range of differences among the states.

1. Only licensed health care providers are protected.
2. Ordinary citizens and licensed providers are protected.
3. Only in-state nurses and physicians are covered.
4. Some states mandate emergency assistance.
5. Others mandate that Good Samaritan laws apply to an emergency at a specific setting, such as at the roadside or outside the workplace.

It is important to know your state's Good Samaritan statutes and adhere to the guidelines in Table 4–3 (Guido, 1997).

▶ TABLE 4–3. GUIDELINES: GOOD SAMARITAN LAWS

1. Make your decision quickly as to whether or not you will stay and help. Remember that there is no common law duty to stop and render aid. Once you begin to provide care, you incur the legal duty to maintain a standard of reasonable emergency care.
2. Ask the injured person or family members for permission to help. Do not force your services if refused.
3. Care for the injured party where you can do so safely. This includes in the vehicle or at the exact site where the victim is found. Move the injured party only if you must do so, without causing further harm and as needed to prevent further harm (eg, off a major highway).
4. Apply the rules of first aid: assess for and prevent bleeding, assess for the need to initiate cardiopulmonary resuscitation, cover the injured party with a blanket or coat, and so forth.
5. Continuously assess and reassess the person for additional injuries, and communicate findings of your assessment to the person or family members.
6. Have someone call or go for additional help while you stay with the injured party.
7. Stay with the person until equally or more qualified help arrives. Prevent unskilled persons from treating or moving the injured party.
8. Give as complete a description as possible of the care that you have rendered to the police and emergency medical personnel so that continuity of care exists. Give family members or police any personal items such as dentures, eyeglasses, and the like.
9. Do not accept any compensation (eg, money or gifts) offered by the injured party or family members. Acceptance of compensation may change your care into a fee-for-service situation and cause you to lose your Good Samaritan protection.
10. Should you choose not to stop and render aid, stop at the nearest phone and report the accident to proper authorities so that the injured party may be aided.
11. Review legislative actions periodically for any changes in your state's Good Samaritan laws. Know the Good Samaritan laws in other states before giving assistance.

Reproduced, with permission, from Guido G. W. (1997). Legal Issues in Nursing, (2nd ed.) Stamford, CT: Appleton & Lange.

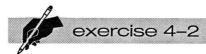

exercise 4-2

Look at your responses to Exercise 4–1. Would you have the same responses after reading the related material in the chapter as you did before?

....

....

....

....

....

If there is a difference, what made the difference?

....

....

....

....

....

How can a shift in your perspective or viewpoint on an issue be of value to you on any issue?

....

....

....

....

....

Malpractice

Only a professional person can be liable for malpractice. A professional person must act in accordance with professional standards that are established by practice boards and professional organizations. If an action is performed by a nonprofessional person that is careless, the result is called "negligence"; the same act performed by a professional person is liability for a malpractice suit (Guido, 1997). The professional person's actions are judged against the prevailing professional standards (Guido, 1997).

There are six elements to be proved in malpractice (Guido, 1997).

1. Duty owed the patient
   A duty of care owed is created by the nurse–patient or provider–patient relationship

2. Breach of the duty owed the patient
   Deviation from the standard of care

3. Foreseeability
   Certain events can be expected to cause certain results

4. Causation
   Injury caused by breach of duty

5. Injury
   Usually physical injuries resulting from breach of duty; emotional injuries must be accompanied by physical injury

6. Damages
   Awarded to assist the injured person in regaining his or her original financial position

Once you are a registered nurse, it is an excellent idea to protect yourself by purchasing professional liability insurance. We are a litigious society and the nature of the practice of nursing makes us vulnerable to malpractice lawsuits. A policy can be purchased for about $100.00 a year, and is tax deductible.

Confidentiality

Webster defines the term "confidential" as "entrusted with private or secret matters, told in confidence." Sensitive information about health status or medical history of individual clients that is not general information is relayed to nurses by either the client or others such as family members and is available through the client's medical record.

Confidentiality is an ethical concept. Any information that is gained as a direct result of the relationship between community based agencies and clients is protected by confidentiality. A breach of confidentiality in this relationship could result in invasion of privacy or a violation of civil law. The staff member responsible for a breach in confidentiality may be held civilly liable for damages and the agency for which the staff member works may be held corporately or vicariously liable (Haddad and Kapp, 1991). In addition, the state licensure act may impose sanctions on both the staff member and agency (Haddad and Kapp, 1991).

There are exceptions to the general confidentiality rule. One is the sharing of information among the interdisciplinary team members who are responsible for the client's care. Written permission for sharing information is usually obtained during the initial visit between the nurse and client. If not, a time-related or event-related release form should be signed for the communication of specific information. This form should include the information to be disclosed, to whom and the time-frame for the release.

In order to receive payment for care, third party payors and insurance companies require certain information about a client's medical diagnosis and the procedures performed in relation to this diagnosis. This confidential information can be released to these parties. Clients may also request information from their records and, even though the actual record is the property of the agency, a copy can be provided. Each agency has policies related to the release of information to clients (Guido, 1997).

REIMBURSEMENT

To reimburse means to be paid for services rendered. Agencies need to be paid for the services they have given to clients.

Medicare, a federal program for those over 65 years of age or disabled, pays billions of dollars each year for the health care of millions of Americans. As the government becomes more and more involved in that health care, the regulations related to the justification of payment for services increase and change. If an agency follows the regulations, payment will follow; if the regulations are not adhered to, payment will be denied.

The written documentation about a specific patient can determine whether or not payment is appropriate. Community based agencies have access to manuals that contain the written regulations that determine eligibility for payment of health care services. The agency is responsible for keeping the staff abreast of new regulations and it is imperative that you learn to accurately document the care you give in a way that supports reimbursement. If the agency is not paid for the care it gives, the agency cannot survive.

The conditions under which Medicare will pay for home care services are (Martinson & Widmer, 1989):

1. The patient is homebound, meaning that the patient's illness or condition makes it very difficult for him or her to leave home. For instance, the patient needs assistance to leave home to keep an appointment at the doctor's office. *Note:* Changes in the criteria for home bound status are in progress.
2. The patient requires skilled services on an intermittent or part-time basis. This is defined by the Health Care Financing Administration as at least one skilled nursing visit in a 60-day period or 2 to 3 visits per week. For a short period, daily visits will be covered. The visits can be made by or supervised by an RN.
3. The physician is responsible for the plan of care. The nurse can develop and coordinate the plan of care, but the physician must approve it.

The types of services covered by Medicare are (Nathanson, 1995):

1. Physical, occupational or speech therapy.
2. Services of a medical social worker who is under the direction of a physician.
3. The part-time services of a home health aide.
4. Medical supplies and durable medical equipment.
5. Medical services provided by an intern or resident of an affiliated approved teaching program.

Medicaid, a program for low income people that is paid for by federal, state, and local money, has patterned its reimbursement requirements after Medicare. Private insurance companies and HMOs also have criteria for payment of health care services. You can now understand the various requirements surrounding reimbursement that the agency demands of its staff. Each nurse could conceivably have to deal with the regulations and required documentation of numerous payors of health care (Medicare, Medicaid, Hospice, insurance companies, and HMOs).

DOCUMENTATION GUIDELINES

Documentation is used for both legal and reimbursement purposes. Nurses have traditionally focused on caring and doing. Documentation, for many years, had been viewed as necessary and approached with reluctance; it was something that had to be done. When you rec-

ognize that the rules an agency has about documentation are to protect the agency and its personnel, you will want to be knowledgeable
about those rules and follow them carefully.

Let's review some of the general rules about documentation that
you have studied and that have legal ramifications. If there is a question about a client's care and the client's record is legible, complete,
and within the standards of care, then you have done your best to protect yourself. The following guidelines must be observed in documenting nursing care:

- Make sure the client's name is on each page of the record
- Date each entry
- Use black or blue ink
- Do not skip lines or leave spaces
- Sign each entry
- Use only agency approved abbreviations

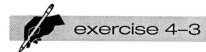 exercise 4–3

Write down several examples of *subjective* statements or
comments that a client may make to you.

Pain in left foot
Itching
Nausea

Write down several examples of *subjective* statements
that a nurse can make in describing a client and/or his environment.

Well-developed, well-nourished
Environment appears safe

- If you make an error, follow the agency's procedures for correcting it (usually marking through the error once with a single line that you date and initial, followed by the correct entry); do not erase or cover with white out
- Never rewrite an entry
- If for some reason there is a delay in writing your notes, put the date and time that you are actually writing the entry, not the date and time you made the visit

Your entries needs to contain objective data. Avoid subjective statements about the client, her family, or environment, especially if there is no accompanying supportive data.

DOCTOR'S ORDERS

Let's take a moment and review a few general rules about doctor's orders and when you need clarification before carrying out doctor's orders.

1. If you are unable to decipher the specific actions involved with the order either on your own or in consulting with other nurses.
2. If you know the order could be harmful to the patient; for example, drug dosages outside of normal limits.
3. If an order goes against the policies or procedures of the agency. An important point to remember is that nurses have the right to refuse to follow through on an order.

If, for whatever reason, you decide not to follow an order as it is written, you must consult with the physician who wrote it and then document it in the client's chart. Follow the chain of command at your agency to report any difficulty with these orders and document it in the client's record.

INCIDENT REPORTS

As human beings, unfortunately, nurses may make mistakes in delivering care and an incident report may need to be completed to record this event. An incident report must be filled out by a professional who comes upon an incident. These reports serve several purposes. The information can be used by agencies to follow through on an incident, such as treating injuries promptly, to identify problem areas that result in staff education, to institute identified preventive measures, and to prepare for litigation, if necessary.

Agencies establish policies to determine the types of incidents to be reported. Familiarize yourself with the agency's regulations about this subject, including the policies and procedures. Ask if you cannot find it in writing.

If an incident does occur, such as a client falling or a medication error, you need to document all the related facts. These facts include:

1. The date and time of the incident; where the incident occurred; and who was notified (by name) at what time; and whether in person or by telephone.

2. Before notifying the physician about the incident, remember to gather the information that will be requested, such as vital signs, name and dosage of a medication, and so on. Document the name of the physician and the time you called her.

3. Document the incident. Do not include the reason why something was inadvertently done or not done; just what occurred. Include any pertinent statements made by the client or family and write them as quotes.

4. In your documentation, include your objective assessments and any actions that you implemented. If you make notes while things are happening, it will be easier to complete the documentation about the incident.

If it becomes evident that an incident report needs to be filed, complete it as directed. As in the hospital setting, you do not write in the client's record that an incident report was completed. Give the report to the appropriate person within the appropriate timeframe. To keep the report confidential, no copies should be made. The agency will store the report in a safe place.

ORIENTATION TO AN AGENCY

Most agencies plan an orientation that is tailored to the needs of the new person. As a student, the type of orientation you receive will depend on the agency. Some agencies are very thorough; others are not. The orientation process is essential for a new staff member. This process is discussed below to assist you as a student and as a graduate nurse.

There are many parts to an orientation and it is important that you are clear about what you need to know so, in the event that it is not made available to you, you can ask. You will meet people in key positions and members of the staff. Take notes as you proceed through this process, including jotting down the names and positions of people you are introduced to either directly or as speakers.

Important issues such as the kind of supervision that can be expected and the availability of a preceptor need to be addressed. You want to seek out the kinds of experiences you are unfamiliar with while you have a preceptor, such as performing a specific procedure. Of course, you must obtain assistance for any aspect of care that you are not comfortable with before giving that care. Inquire about the chain of command in the agency and know who to contact first if you need assistance or have to report specific information.

The agency's philosophy, mission statement, and objectives are statements about the agency's beliefs and goals. During the orientation process, these documents will be made available to you; if they are not provided, you need to ask to see them. After carefully reading these documents, you will know if your beliefs and goals are compatible with those of the agency. You will understand the direction the agency is taking, how resources are allocated, and how the agency will support you.

In order to have a comprehensive picture of what the nurse is expected to be and do for an agency, there are several written documents that need your close attention during your orientation. These documents come from different sources; however, they are linked together to form what constitutes the basis for nursing practice. We will consider each of these documents so you understand their interrelatedness.

First there is the **job description.** For each position that an agency fills, there is a corresponding job description. As a student, you can practice becoming familiar with this document. Study the job description for the registered nurse at the agency in which you are assigned to your clinical experiences. The job description presents the parameters, responsibilities, and expectations of the position. Can you fulfill what the description demands?

In addition to the job description, a set of agency policies and procedures, which are usually contained in large notebooks, are available during orientation. You need to carefully study these **policies and procedures.** The word "study" is used deliberately because you must be familiar with these documents so as to protect yourself. Note the wording of the statements. Do you feel comfortable with the wording? You need to know the location of these documents so you can review them whenever you have a question or want to verify something. If any of these documents is omitted from the orientation, it is your responsibility to ask to see them.

At this point, we need to focus on the **Nurse Practice Act.** Each state has its own Nurse Practice Act that has been passed by that state's legislature. This document is law. The Nurse Practice Act is available from the State Board of Nursing for the state in which you will be practicing nursing. It is imperative that you obtain a copy and be thoroughly aware of all its provisions. Remember to periodically request an updated copy.

In addition to the Nurse Practice Act, you need to be familiar with the **standards of care** for the specialty of nursing you are practicing. The American Nurses Association has developed standards of practice for many nursing specialties and various professional organi-

 exercise 4–4

Do this exercise with the students in your clinical group (6–10 students). Divide the group into equal subgroups. Each subgroup is assigned to obtain one or more of the following documents from the agencies in which you are assigned for your clinical experiences (except the policies and procedures). Study your assigned documents:

1. The agency's philosophy
2. Mission statement
3. Objectives
4. Job description
5. Nurse Practice Act for your state
6. Standards of Care for the specialty of nursing you will be practicing (hospice nursing, home health nursing, occupational nursing, and so on)

The policies and procedures are usually in one or more large books that you can review in the agency, but not remove. In other words, you cannot receive a copy of this document. However, you can review its contents and take notes so you know the type of material that it contains.

After gathering and studying your assigned materials, meet as a total group. Distribute the documents and discuss them as a group.

zations have also developed standards of care for their specialty areas. Thoroughly read the standards of practice that apply to the area in which you plan to practice.

All of these documents (the job description, policies and procedures, the Nurse Practice Act, and standards of care for the specialty) are important to your nursing practice. If there is a question about the care that a client received, the practice of the nurse involved is measured against the content of these documents. The standards of care described in these materials represent the practice of an average or reasonably prudent nurse. Familiarity with the contents of these documents facilitates the nurse's adherence to the boundaries that constitute safe nursing care. This care includes knowing the tasks that can be delegated to untrained assistants, the situations in which the physician must be notified, the guidelines for teaching the client or caregiver about a specific procedure or medical equipment that must be maintained, and the appropriate documentation.

THE INTERDISCIPLINARY HEALTH CARE TEAM

Many community based agencies use the expertise of various disciplines through the use of interdisciplinary teams. As the needs of the client become evident, a member of this team can be called on to assess specific areas of the client's life and assist with care. The quality of care provided to clients is dependent on the people who deliver that care. A team that is multidisciplinary and well-coordinated increases the resources available to both the nurse and the client.

Your orientation to an agency includes the composition of its team. The team may consist of the following professionals and non-professionals.

Nurse

The nurse plays a vital role as a member of the interdisciplinary team and is often the professional who has the most contact with the client, particularly over time. The addition of new team members to the client's interdisciplinary team is often the result of needs and problems identified by the nurse. Frequently, the nurse is the case manager for the client and thus coordinates the client's care, including scheduling team meetings.

Physician

The role of the physician can vary from agency to agency. As you would expect, physicians are responsible for doctor's orders in all settings. In addition to medical orders, the physician is responsible for the plan of care in home care settings. Some physicians are very involved in the client's plan of care whereas others depend heavily on the nurses within the agency. Either way, the physician must approve the plan of care.

Social Worker

A social worker focuses on the psychosocial adjustments of the client and family to illness and can assess the home for safety and for the appropriateness of various types of home care. A referral for the services of a social worker, in home care, must be prescribed by a physician and included in the physician's plan of care so as to be reimbursable by Medicare and Medicaid. At this time, medical social work is not considered to be a skilled service by these payors.

The social worker develops a plan of care with the client and family after an assessment has been completed. An essential part of this plan is teaching coping skills through counseling to help them maintain equilibrium during illness. There is a focus on referring and linking the client to necessary community resources, such as the delivery of meals. The social worker also functions as an advocate, a mediator, and a collaborator. The level of care needed by a person, whether it be long-term care or assistance in the home, is often determined by this assessment (Sar and Phillips, 1997).

Physical Therapist

The physical therapist is a licensed rehabilitation specialist who focuses on physical fitness and mobility. The purpose of physical therapy (PT) is to promote optimal health and functional independence in people with health problems resulting from disease or injury.

The goal of the physical therapist is to alleviate acute and chronic movement dysfunction, pain, or physical disability. This is accomplished by assessing functional limitations, impairments, and disability through examination. A diagnosis, interventions, and prognosis are then determined (Miller-Keane, 1997). Interventions may include appropriate exercise such as range of motion, stretching and strengthening of muscles, the application of heat and cold, and the teaching of self-care techniques.

Most physical therapists practice in community-based settings; approximately 30% practice in hospitals (Miller-Keane, 1997).

Occupational Therapist

Occupational therapy (OT) is one of the fastest growing health care fields. It is the science and practice of activities of daily living such as eating, playing, working, self-care, and caring for others and the immediate environment. The goal of occupational therapy is the development and maintenance of the capacity to perform roles and tasks essential to productive living to the satisfaction of self and others.

The occupational therapist evaluates and treats problems that reduce a client's ability to cope with the tasks of everyday living. These problems can be of a developmental, physical, emotional, or social nature. The interventions of the occupational therapist increase performance capacity and facilitate the development of adaptive skills (Miller-Keane, 1997).

Enterostomal Therapist

Enterostomal therapy (ET) includes care of clients with ostomies, wound care, and continence nursing practice. An enterostomal therapist specializes in skin and wound care associated with the presence of an enterostomy. In addition, the enterostomal therapist assesses and establishes a plan of care to manage ostomies, skin problems, complex wounds, and fistulas. These interventions include the fitting of prosthetic equipment for ostomies, giving emotional support to clients and families, and educating staff, clients, and caregivers about issues related to skin care.

Dietitian

The goal of the dietitian is the promotion of health through proper diet. In the presence of disease or other disorders, the dietitian is responsible for the therapeutic use of diet in treatment (Miller-Keane, 1997).

The services of a dietitian may be needed on a periodic basis in various community-based settings. This situation leads to contractual agreements between a dietitian and an agency that are applied when questions arise or if the nurse needs guidance in planning the care for a specific client.

Chaplain or Other Spiritual Advisors

Spiritual care is needed whenever there is evidence of the client experiencing spiritual distress related to illness or disability. The nurse who listens intently to the client can recognize the opportunity to assist with questions and doubts related to spiritual issues and to give support and encouragement. Referral to a chaplain or spiritual advisor of choice is important. Unfortunately, however, a referral is often the result of the degree of involvement of the health care professional in the client's spiritual problems or issues. The nurse needs to be sensitive to the client's verbal and non-verbal expressions about this aspect of his or her life in order to provide the necessary support.

Chaplains play an integral role on hospice interdisciplinary teams and in acute care settings. Their role in other community based settings is usually on a referral basis (Miller-Keane, 1997).

Communication Among Team Members

Team members record pertinent data in the client's chart after their visits or appointments with a client. Usually there is a specific area in the chart designated for each professional's entry. Even though health care professionals have access to each other's notations about the client, interpersonal communication is necessary to fully support client goals. Interdisciplinary team meetings provide an excellent avenue for the exchange of pertinent information.

Listen carefully to the client information disclosed during these meetings; it often reveals significant data about the client that has not been previously recorded in the client's record. For instance, there may be extensive discussion about each client's family life and the impact illness has on this structure, but this information may not be entered on the flow sheets or other forms in the chart. Interdisciplinary team meetings provide the opportunity for sharing information that is helpful in understanding family dynamics, life style, and client interactions. This is the time to ask questions or clarify information about the plan of care. Participate in the discussions. The knowledge you accumulate can be very valuable in your nursing practice because what you learn while caring for one client can often be applied in another situation.

Developing and maintaining good rapport with each of the members of the interdisciplinary team can be of immeasurable value because you will be able to use this knowledge throughout your career. An example is attending sessions between the physical therapist and a client in which range of motion exercises are being taught. You can observe how the therapist holds an extremity during an exercise and listen to the instructions being given to a family member.

Supervision of Non-Professional Workers

Non-professionals, such as nursing aides, nursing assistants, and volunteers, play a major role in the care of clients for a variety of agencies. The level of care that the non-professional is engaged in directly influences the type of supervision needed. For example, a volunteer who helps a client by writing a dictated letter needs a different type of supervision than a home care aide who provides total care to a bedridden client.

Nurses must understand that they are responsible for the care given by non-professionals, untrained assistants, or caregivers. The nurse needs to ensure that a nursing assistant is able to safely provide care to the client and has sufficient training for assigned tasks. If there are any questions or "hunches" that the care delivered by a non-professional worker may not meet prescribed nursing standards, the nurse must investigate the situation. The assistant is asked to demonstrate the skill that is in question to make sure that correct procedural technique is being used. The findings need to be documented carefully.

MEDIATION OF CONFLICTS

In community based settings, nurses are in a position to be informed about various kinds of conflicts involving clients, caregivers, team members, and others. In these situations, the following guidelines can assist you in establishing and maintaining open communication.

1. Put your feelings aside and be objective about the situation.
2. Listen carefully to what is being presented.
3. Keep in mind that the client's health care needs are primary.
4. If the conflict involves you, state your position clearly by using "I" rather than "you."
5. Have one person speak at a time and clarify what is being said if necessary.
6. Identify possible options.
7. If a serious problem exists, consider recommending an appropriate source of assistance whether it be the administrative personnel of your agency or a community agency.

8. In every conflict, people have different perspectives on the same issue. Accept and appreciate each person's position.

Conflicts, when managed skillfully, present the opportunity for creative solutions to problems. The quality of care provided to clients increases and staff and agency goals are strengthened.

COMMUNITY RESOURCES

Community resources are those services provided by public or private agencies or organizations at little or no cost. A **public agency** is one that is supported by tax money from the federal, state, or local level or any combination of the three. Examples of public agencies are a Department of Social Services, a Department of Health, and a Rural Health Clinic.

A **private agency** is one that is funded by private sources, donations and/or payment for their services. There are two types of private agencies:

1. *Non-profit.* Refers to tax exempt status; examples of non-profit agencies are the United Way, the American Heart Association and churches.
2. *For profit.* Many home care agencies are structured as for-profit agencies.

Available Resources

The resources present in one community differ from those of another. It is important to be aware of the available services in your area and to know how to locate a needed service.

Identification of Needs

Community resources are needed when an individual or family has the potential of or is having difficulty managing their lives. In our society, we tend to wait until a problem occurs before we take action. This response can be considered as secondary and tertiary prevention. As a nurse, you are able to help clients participate in primary prevention activities, even though this intervention may not be a required component of the plan of care. This activity takes time and, remember, you cannot accurately measure the outcome of primary prevention because the event may or may not have happened without the intervention.

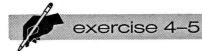

exercise 4–5

This is a clinical group exercise. Each group member works on one of the following:

1. Is there a directory or a publication that describes the services available in the community? Where does one obtain a copy? Does it cost anything? Obtain a copy for student reference.

....

....

....

....

....

....

2. Are there agencies such as United Way? Which organizations benefit from this agency? Obtain a list.

....

....

....

....

....

....

3. Are there community services available in a nearby rural county (if applicable)? Do agencies in the surrounding areas offer any services to residents in the rural county?

....

....

....

....

....

....

4. Are other sources—for example, the public library, media, recorded messages for various conditions or diseases—available? If yes, obtain information.

....

....

....

....

....

5. Is any information available on the Internet? If so, write a summary for your classmates.

....

....

....

....

....

6. Is transportation available to those who have no transportation? If so, what are the criteria and rules for use?

....

....

....

....

....

....

7. Put together a system for filing and storing the above gathered information for future student and faculty use.

....

....

....

....

....

Your continuous assessment of your client's condition provides clues as to the types of resources needed at a given point in time. Your interaction with the client and caregiver further defines their needs and determines the appropriateness of introducing additional resources.

THE REFERRAL PROCESS

The referral process is a systematic problem-solving approach involving actions that assist the client to use resources that can hopefully resolve his needs. The success of this process depends on open communication and the exchange of information. The role of the nurse in the referral process includes the following elements:

- Introducing the client to the resource
- Clarifying expectations
- Facilitating the coordination of care to be provided

Basic Principles of the Referral Process

The principles of the referral process are similar to those that form the basis of the nursing process and are discussed below.

- Assessment
  Establish a working relationship with the client.
  Assess the need for a referral.
- Planning
  Set objectives for the referral.
- Implementation
  Explore available resources.
  Acknowledge the client's decision about accepting or not accepting the referral.
  If appropriate, make the referral to the resource.
  If possible, the client/family makes the initial contact to a resource; it has been found that the client is more likely to follow through on the referral if she takes the initiative. However, this action may not be feasible depending on the client's situation. *Note:* A consent form must be signed by the client before any records are sent to another agency or organization.
  Facilitate the client's access to the resource by writing down and discussing:
  The time of the appointment
  The address of the agency
  The contact person
  Any needed directions

- Evaluation and follow up
    Maintain confidentiality during the entire process.
    Assign primary responsibility for nursing care to one agency
        to avoid fragmentation.
    Evaluate the complete and specific information transmitted
        between agencies.
    Document and maintain records.
    Perform quality assurance as it relates to access to care,
        outcome criteria, and cost-effectiveness of interventions.

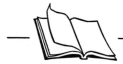

CHAPTER HIGHLIGHTS

1. Knowledge of ethical and legal issues for nurses in general alerts you to areas of potential liability in community based practice.

2. The rules and regulations for reimbursement need to be followed to ensure payment for services provided by community based agencies.

3. Knowledge about the procedures involved with documentation, doctor's orders, and how incident reports protect the nurse.

4. Grouped together, the job description of a specific position, policies and procedures of an agency, the Nurse Practice Act, and standards of care provide the components of acceptable nursing practice.

5. The interdisciplinary health care team plays a major role in client care.

6. The management of conflict is vital to the well-being of the client and quality of nursing care.

7. Application of knowledge of community resources and the referral process is a primary function of the community based nurse.

REFERENCES

Guido, G.W. (1997). *Legal Issues in Nursing.* (2nd ed.) Stamford, CT: Appleton & Lange.

Haddad, A.M. & Kapp, M.B. (1991). *Ethical and Legal Issues in Home Health Care.* Stamford, CT: Appleton & Lange.

Martinson, I. & Widmer, A. (1989). *Home Health Nursing Care.* Philadelphia: Saunders.

Miller-Keane. (1997). *Encyclopedia & Dictionary of Medicine, Nursing, & Allied Health.* (6th ed.) Philadelphia: Saunders.

Nathanson, M.D. (1995). *Home Health Care Answer Book: Legal Issues for Providers.* Rockville, MD: Aspen.

Sar, B.K. & Phillips, I. (1997). The role of the social worker in home care. In: Spratt, J.S., Hawley, R.L., & Hoye, R. (Eds.): *Home Health Care.* Delray Beach, FL: St. Lucie Press.

III.

KNOWLEDGE APPLICABLE TO COMMUNITY BASED NURSING

5.

Cultural Diversity

 exercise 5–1

List cultural practices, traditions, behaviors and/or ways of thinking that originate from your culture(s) of origin that have survived in your family.

1. ....

2. ....

3. ....

4. ....

5. ....

In community based nursing, you will have the opportunity to put into practice what you have learned thus far about cultural diversity from nursing and sociology courses. **Cultural diversity** "refers to the variations and differences among and between cultural groups due to differences in lifeways, language, values, norms and other cutural aspects" (Leininger, 1995, p. 69).

Remember, the lifestyle of patients in the hospital may be viewed as irrelevant or unnecessary for the care and treatments given within the institution. In this setting, the nurse gets only glimpses into who the patient is: age, color, certain habits, foreign or regional accent, birthplace, and the amount of care received for the condition or disease. Judgments that are inaccurate and unjust to the patient are often made from this incredibly small amount of data.

In community based nursing, the nurse receives a full view of the client's lifestyle. The greater the difference in lifestyles between the nurse and the client, the easier it is to make quick judgments. An awareness of this fact can remind you to withhold any judgments as you focus your attention on the client and his family as they reveal who they are to you. It is a great privilege to be invited into people's lives to assist them with their health care needs. Knowledge of cultural diversity is important because if or when certain cultural aspects surface that demonstrate a difference in perspective, you will have some understanding and appreciate those differences.

CONCEPTS RELATED TO CULTURE

As a review, you know that culture is dynamic, learned, shared, and integrated into the lives of people. Culture is such a part of us that we are most often unaware of how it affects us. This characteristic makes it easier to identify cultural aspects in others rather than in ourselves. A member of one culture can no more experience another culture from the inside than a male or female can experience being the opposite sex.

It can be helpful to observe culture from the standpoint of beliefs because the subject of culture is extremely complex. Included in the beliefs that people hold are those derived from the person's culture of origin. These beliefs permeate thoughts and actions and influence variables such as practices, rituals, customs, habits, likes and dislikes, and lifestyles. These collective beliefs are extremely powerful, and the violation of any one of them can result in collective sanctions.

There are times when sanctions are imposed on you and there are times when you may impose sanctions on others. Most of the time, people are unaware of this behavior.

There are cultures within cultures. The formation of these groups can be related to geographic influences that cause differences in speech patterns, behavior, and viewpoints. For example, different sections of our country (south, west, north, and east) have an effect on the people who live there. It is not until one is immersed in another section of our country that the differences become obvious.

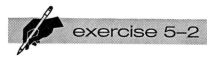

exercise 5–2

Think about the religion you belong to and one of the most important holidays. An example: Christian/Christmas. Suppose you decided not to celebrate Christmas in any way. What do you think might be some of the reactions of your family, friends and others?

....
....
....
....
....
....
....

How would you feel?

....
....
....
....
....
....
....

Would these reactions or sanctions lead you to continue observance of the tradition?

....
....
....
....
....
....

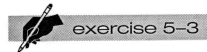

exercise 5-3

When you see an interracial couple together, one from your race and one from another, what are your thoughts?

....

....

....

....

....

Would you feel differently if the person who is of your race is the opposite sex from you?

....

....

....

....

....

Changes do occur in cultures over time. For example, not too many years ago, smoking in our culture was totally acceptable. People smoked everywhere and ashtrays or other containers were readily available. Even doctors smoked publicly. However, changes in what we believe about smoking resulted in changes related to where people are permitted to smoke. If you step into another culture where smoking is acceptable and there are no restrictions on where people can smoke, you will experience "culture shock."

Knowledge about other cultures and how intricately woven culture is in the lives of its members can give nurses important insights about their clients and why they may be behaving in certain ways. The farther the client's culture is from your own, the less likely you are to understand the client's behavior. Even if you lived in another culture, there would still be subtleties of culture that you would never grasp due to not being an integral part of that culture.

Ethnocentrism "refers to the belief that one's own ways are the best, most superior, or preferred to act, believe, or behave" (Leininger, 1995, p.65). Many health care professionals approach the lifestyle changes that would be in the client's best interest from this perspective. This attitude may lead nurses to honestly believe that these changes are essential for the client to make and that there is no possibility of compromise. Clients who do not make the changes are labelled as being noncompliant. Ethnocentrism that involves the health care professional imposing his or her professional beliefs on the patient or client is known as **cultural imposition.**

 exercise 5–4

Recall a time when you were struggling with a life issue.

1. Feel what it felt like to have another judge you at that point.

   ....

   ....

   ....

   ....

   ....

2. Feel what it felt like when another provided you the space to be where you were and reached out to you.

   ....

   ....

   ....

   ....

   ....

3. Describe the difference between the two.

   ....

   ....

   ....

   ....

   ....

In caring for clients and proposing changes in lifestyle, such as diet, exercise, and other practices, it can be valuable to remember how entrenched these aspects of living are in the client's life. It is difficult enough to make life changes when one wants to make those changes. These changes present challenges to the client and to the nurse as they work together. A willingness on the part of the client to change usually encourages the nurse. The situation is completely different if the client has no desire to alter anything. The resistance from the client can be very discouraging. The nurse in a community based setting who is less likely to experience "burn-out" in this situation is the one who is able to be compassionate by releasing judgments, expectations, and a need to control.

If we approach cultural diversity from the position of collective beliefs combined with individual beliefs, it becomes clear that superimposing generalizations on a member of a cultural group just because she is a member of that group is unfair. Not everyone adheres to the collective beliefs of their culture of origin; some beliefs may be held and others changed. Expecting certain cultural aspects to be present only because the person is from a certain culture introduces judgments that may be grossly inaccurate. It is crucial to accept people as you find them without stereotyping or superimposing a cultural template on them just because they are from a specific culture. **Stereotyping** "is the assumption that all people in a similar cultural, racial, or ethnic group are alike and share the same values and beliefs" (Giger & Davidhizar, 1995, p.65). Judgments about cultural beliefs or practices are communicated on both the intuitive and non-verbal levels; in other words, not a word needs to be spoken for these attitudes to be clearly transmitted.

DOMINANT AND MINORITY CULTURES

A dominant culture is not necessarily dominant because of the number of people in that group, just as a minority culture does not always have fewer numbers than the dominant culture. A dominant culture is one that has power, guards the value system, and may even designate who are the minorities. An example of this can be found in the American workplace. In this environment, males are members of the dominant culture and females form the minority culture. Females are often underrepresented in upper management and the males, who dominate management, have the power to perpetuate this situation.

A minority group is kept in the minority because of its powerlessness. Cultural minorities are considered to be inferior, without power,

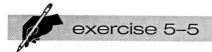

exercise 5-5

A student from the North arrived in a southern town to attend graduate school. Within a few hours of her arrival, someone called her a "damned Yankee." This took her by surprise. Later she realized that if you lose something, like a war, you never forget it. If you win, you forget about it. Because the North won the Civil War, the entire issue was not a part of her, yet that one expression made her feel separate.

Have you ever had something projected onto you just because you are a member of a specific group (race, age, sex, location, etc.)?

....
....
....
....
....

Have you ever done this to another person?

....
....
....
....
....

What makes the difference between including or seperating another person from your perspective?

....
....
....
....
....
....

and may have undesireable characteristics (Giger and Davidhizar, 1995).

A member of the dominant culture does not have to concern himself with what it means to be different or deal with various forms of discrimination on a continuous basis. If you are a nurse from the dominant culture, it is important to be aware of this as you work with members of a cultural minority.

CULTURAL PHENOMENA

There are six cultural phenomena that are present in all cultures (Giger & Davidhizar, 1995). They are: (1) communication, (2) space, (3) social organization, (4) time orientation, (5) environmental control, and (6) biological variations. Assessment of each of these areas facilitates the interconnectedness of culture and nursing practice. Figure 5–1 includes a range of specific data within each category of phenomena that is vital to a cultural assessment.

In Table 5–1, five cultures are viewed in terms of the six cultural phenomena. Studying these criteria can make you aware of the vast differences among cultures and help you to be culturally sensitive.

SPECIFIC ISSUES RELATED TO CULTURAL DIVERSITY

There are specific issues or paradigms that need to be addressed in and of themselves because they are not limited to a specific culture. Two of these issues are the effects of poverty on well-being and health, and the influence of nontraditional practices on health care.

Poverty

Members of every cultural group can be affected by poverty. In 1964, the Department of Health, Education and Welfare (HEW) (now the Department of Health and Human Services [DHHS]) developed guidelines to determine eligibility for monetary assistance for people below specific income levels. These guidelines change annually and are based on the Consumer Price Index. The 1995 guideline for poverty was $15,150 for a family of four (Federal Registry, 1995). Each

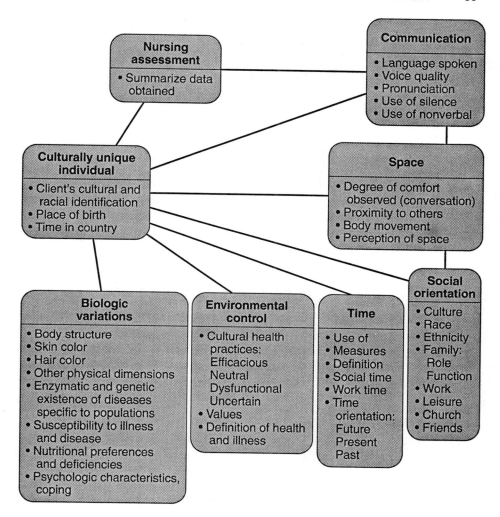

Figure 5–1. Assessment of clients via cultural phenomena. *Reprinted with permission from Giger, J. and Davidhizar, R. (1995). Transcultural Nursing: Assessment and Intervention. (2nd Ed.) St. Louis: Mosby.*

state has the option of adding to but not subtracting from this figure when determining eligibility for a specific program.

The government, over recent years, has developed numerous programs to assist those in poverty. In the process of "helping" people, we often unknowingly diminish their personal power. **Each time you give someone something, you take something away.** To illustrate, an impoverished single mother at the turn of the century had to be cre-

▶ TABLE 5-1. CROSS-CULTURAL EXAMPLES OF CULTURAL PHENOMENA

Nations of Origin	Communication	Space	Time Orientation	Social Organization	Environmental Control	Biological Variations
Asian China Hawaii Philippines Korea Japan Southeast Asia (Laos, Cambodia, Vietnam)	National language preference Dialects, written characters Use of silence Nonverbal and contextual cuing	Noncontact people	Present	Family: hierarchical structure, loyalty Devotion to tradition Many religions, including Taoism, Buddhism, Islam, and Christianity Community social organizations	Traditional health and illness beliefs Use of traditional medicines Traditional practitioners: Chinese doctors and herbalists	Liver cancer Stomach cancer Coccidioidomycosis Hypertension Lactose intolerance
African West Coast (as slaves) Many African countries West Indian Islands Dominican Republic Haiti Jamaica	National languages Dialect: Pidgin, Creole, Spanish, and French	Close personal space	Present over future	Family: many female, single parent Large, extended family networks Strong church affiliation within community Community social organizations	Traditional health and illness beliefs Folk medicine tradition Traditional healer: root-worker	Sickle cell anemia Hypertension Cancer of the esophagus Stomach cancer Coccidioidomycosis Lactose intolerance

Origin	Communication	Space	Time Orientation	Social Organization	Health Beliefs	High-Risk Health Problems
Europe Germany England Italy Ireland Other European countries	National languages Many learn English immediately	Noncontact people Aloof Distant Southern countries: closer contact and touch	Future over present	Nuclear families Extended families Judeo-Christian religions Community social organizations	Primary reliance on modern health care system Traditional health and illness beliefs Some remaining folk medicine traditions	Breast cancer Heart disease Diabetes mellitus Thalassemia
Native American 170 Native American tribes Aleuts Eskimos	Tribal languages Use of silence and body language	Space very important and has no boundaries	Present	Extremely family oriented Biological and extended families Children taught to respect traditions Community social organizations	Traditional health and illness beliefs Folk medicine tradition Traditional healer: medicine man	Accidents Heart disease Cirrhosis of the liver Diabetes mellitus
Hispanic countries Spain Cuba Mexico Central and South America	Spanish or Portuguese primary language	Tactile relationships Touch Handshakes Embracing Value physical presence	Present	Nuclear family Extended families *Compadrazzo:* godparents Community social organizations	Traditional health and illness beliefs Folk medicine tradition Traditional healers: *Curandero, Espiritista, Partera, Señora*	Diabetes mellitus Parasites Coccidioidomycosis Lactose intolerance

From Spector, RE. (1996). Guide to Heritage Assessment and Health Traditions. Stamford, CT: Appleton & Lange, pp. 8–10.

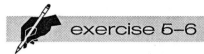

exercise 5–6

Have you and your family ever been in poverty? Have you found a way out of this condition or have you been able to view poverty from a distance?

....

....

....

....

....

My beliefs about poverty are:

1. ....

2. ....

3. ....

4. ....

ative and resourceful in the struggle to feed, clothe, and shelter her family with little or no public assistance. This process, no matter how tedious, supported her ability to manage her family's existence.

In contrast, the life of the single mother of today is quite different. She has access to numerous federal and state assistance programs that provide most of the direction of her family's life. This mother does not need to worry about paying the rent because public housing and utilities are paid by the Aid to Families with Dependent Children (AFDC) program. The provision of food for her family is not a concern either; breakfast and lunch are provided at school through free programs. In addition, food stamps and The Women, Infants and Children (WIC) programs also provide free food. If her children become ill, she takes them to a physician knowing that Medicaid will pay the bill for the medical care and for any needed medications.

In the process of helping families in poverty, all of the above programs have created a life of subsistence; a culture of poverty. The subtle trade-off for receiving these services is the relinquishment of any or all management skills of the mother and ultimately those of her children. As a result, generations of people who are unable to manage

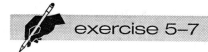

exercise 5-7

What do you think a family receiving federal and state assistance for generations would believe about themselves when faced with various cuts in benefits?

1. ....
2. ....
3. ....
4. ....
5. ....

What do you think the people in elected office who need to cut assistance programs believe about those in poverty?

1. ....
2. ....
3. ....

their own lives are vulnerable to politically-based program cuts and new paradigms such as managed care and capitation. Because of this situation, many of them are helpless and feel hopeless.

As you assess the client and his family who live in poverty, listen to what they say to identify the beliefs they hold about themselves and their circumstances. Any sense of lack of control over their lives can greatly affect their ability to take initiative in caring for themselves and in following directions. Concentrate on the most important nursing measure that needs to be implemented, taking one step at a time. Remember, we tend to view the world through our own experiences. In other words, it is easy to make the assumption that someone is able to read and write, has a pen or pencil and paper, and is able to keep a record of a task or action needed for an assessment. This may not be the case.

Nontraditional Health Practices in the United States

A new paradigm that first originated in the 1970s has lately been gaining increasing prominence in our mainstream culture. This paradigm centers on wellness, fitness, and nontraditional modalities of treatment. It has become more visible through books, magazine and journal articles, television programs, and increased numbers of health food stores. In response to this attention from the general public, a full range of nontraditional practices with a holistic focus has emerged. They include both the expansion of practices that have been available for many years such as homeopathy, chiropractic, and naturopathy, as well as other practices that are new to Americans, some of which originated from other cultures and others that were developed by individuals. These practices include Reiki, yoga, acupuncture, acupressure, reflexology, massage therapy, and healing touch. Lay people learned they could take responsibility for their well-being by involving themselves in fitness programs, eating natural foods, and practicing imagery and meditation.

 exercise 5–8

At a Fall 1996 professional conference on lactation in Chapel Hill, North Carolina (The Art of Breastfeeding: Working Together to Make Breastfeeding a Success), a physician lectured on herbs, with dosages, that support lactation. Relaxation, imagery, breast massage, use of music, and breath work were also discussed.

What do you think most physicians' opinions about these modalities would be?

....

....

....

....

....

How would you get them to change their opinions?

....

....

....

....

....

In our culture, we use the terms "health" and "sickness" interchangeably. The term "health care system" is used when we really mean "sick care system" and we pay for "health insurance" that we use when we are sick (Armentrout, 1993). The term "wellness" is often used to eliminate the confusion that surrounds the term health.

As with any new paradigm, nontraditional paradigms were initially rejected by both medicine and nursing. A **paradigm shifter** is the person who develops a new paradigm and **paradigm pioneers** are the small number of followers of the new paradigm (Barker, 1997). An example of a paradigm shifter in nursing is Delores Krieger. She developed Therapeutic Touch, a modality that was introduced into the medical system in the 1970s. A small number of nurses were courageous pioneers and nurtured the new modality. Today, therapeutic touch is widely taught and practiced in nursing. The same situation occurred with wellness and holistic paradigms in medicine. Physicians Deepak Chopra (1990) and Dean Ornish (1993) were paradigm shifters when they published their nontraditional works. Their ideas began to permeate the health care system and are beginning to become tolerable to the majority of health care professionals.

As you practice in community based nursing, you may care for clients who subscribe to nontraditional paradigms. Open your mind and listen, especially to evidence of this paradigm permeating professional practice and literature. An example is Oxford Health Plans Inc., of Norwalk, Connecticut, one of the nation's largest HMOs, which has approved the inclusion of 1000 credentialed naturopathic doctors, chiropractors, acupuncturists, and other alternative practitioners in their provider lists as of January 1, 1997. As a result, clients do not need primary care physician pre-approval for these visits, which means these holistic practitioners bypass the gatekeepers. In addition, Oxford has a division that sells medicinal herbs (Lagnado, 1996).

Cultural Assessment

A cultural assessment of a client and family is extremely valuable to the nurse in community based nursing. The physical data related to a client's illness can lead to an accurate nursing care plan; whether or not the plan is successfully implemented, however, can depend on the integration of aspects of the cultural assessment. The first part of a cultural assessment consists of a self assessment of your cultural beliefs. Assessing your own culture is a continuous process and bringing certain beliefs to your awareness takes time.

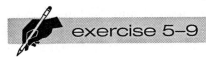 exercise 5–9

Step back and observe your own family as if from a distance, without judgment. Which group of people does your family make negative statements about?

....

....

....

....

....

Where do you think they got those beliefs?

....

....

....

....

....

Would you ever bring someone of that group home to dinner with you?

....

....

....

....

....

If you did, what do you think would happen?

....

....

....

....

....

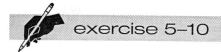
exercise 5–10

When a person has said or done something to you that greatly upsets you, how do you do usually handle it?

Work at identifying what has "hooked" you. An example: Two friends, one normal weight, the other overweight, were having lunch together. They both ordered the same dessert. As the waitress approached she scanned the overweight person, looked at the desserts and gave her the smaller dessert even though the larger dessert was in the waitress' closer hand. This action infuriated the overweight friend.

The obvious reason for her anger appeared to be the fact that she got the smaller dessert. But, upon analysis, it became apparent that the real issue was that the waitress looked at her size, made a judgment, and then acted on that judgment by giving her the smaller dessert. Anytime this young lady encountered someone making a hasty judgment and acting upon it, she would have had the same reaction.

Now that the real issue has been brought to her awareness, the young lady is instantly aware of what the other person is doing and she no longer reacts, although she may choose to respond.

Some of your most important realizations about yourself and your attitudes towards others can happen while you are caring for clients of a different culture. Stay alert to the various feelings that surface as you are practicing. These feelings will usually take you by surprise. When things are going along smoothly, it can be a sign that we are not learning too much. When someone or something irritates or annoys you, it is a signal that, if you choose, you can learn about yourself.

Conducting a cultural assessment of a client takes time. The first step of this process is to establish a trusting relationship. In community based nursing, the nurse usually works with the client over a period of time, which proves to be an advantage because it allows for an on-going collection of information about cultural beliefs and practices. As your client and her family realize and accept that you are there to assist them, not to judge, then a working relationship can be established.

In your initial work-up of the client, you will need to collect specific information. The exact format in which this information is recorded depends on your agency and the forms you are required to use. Some of that information is related to culture, such as religious preference, ethnic background, support system, food preferences, health practices, and family structure and patterns. Obtaining this data through informal conversation can be more effective than asking a continuous stream of questions. This data is then integrated into your nursing practice by planning, implementing, and evaluating the influences of culture. If you know and respect what the client believes about his condition or disease and how he lives, you can create a plan of care that will not only have meaning for the client and family members but that could be more effective.

A generalization to keep in mind as you begin your cultural assessment is that socioeconomic level can greatly influence which health practices are followed. Those in lower socioeconomic groups tend to follow traditional or folk health systems, while those in higher socioeconomic classes may also practice traditional remedies while questioning their basis or value. Members of wealthy socioeconomic classes tend to use scientific medicine (Clark, 1996).

Know the cultural groups in your area who could potentially be clients. Your goal is to become culturally competent by knowing all you can about the prevalent culture and even studying the language. If your client's first language is not English, observe the nonverbal body language, expressions, motions, and gestures that will give you clues as to whether or not the person understands your words. If something does not seem to fit, check it out. Keep in mind that if the client speaks some English and you are trying to assess if he understands you, the tendency is to raise the volume of your voice. Remember, the client is not having difficulty hearing; he does not understand the words. Instead of raising your voice, slowly repeat or reword what you said.

Know the resources in your community, particularly those related to the services of an interpreter or translator if needed. Observe the following guidelines when considering the use of these professionals.

- Before engaging a translator, make sure the language is compatible for dialect and regional differences.
- When interacting with a client and translator, speak slowly and avoid expressions that are metaphors or slang.
- Using family members as translators or interpreters can be difficult for the client if the discussion of a particular illness is

sensitive for the client. The same is true with involving members of the opposite sex as translators.

- Confidentiality may be threatened if the translator knows the client or is from the same community.

Departments may be available on the state level that offer support to those of different cultures. For example, there may be a telephone number for health care professionals to call to obtain health-related terminology in a specific language. On the local level, there may be agencies, clubs, and organizations that can be of assistance in helping you provide culturally sensitive care.

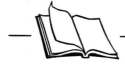

CHAPTER HIGHLIGHTS

1. Knowledge about a specific culture can lead to understanding when cultural influences present themselves. However, there is a very fine line between using this knowledge to help you and stereotyping the individual.

2. Knowledge of cultural diversity can lead to accurate assessments of a client, family, and community.

3. Assess each person for who they are.

4. Information about the dominant culture, cultural minorities, and cultural phenomena need to be included in a culturally sensitive assessment.

5. Poverty and nontraditional health practices can be present in any cultural group.

6. A thorough cultural assessment, conducted over time, provides the most accurate information about cultural issues relevant to the client and his significant others.

REFERENCES

Armentrout, G. (1993). A comparison of the medical model and the wellness model. *Journal of Holistic Nursing* 7:57.

Barker, J. (1997). *Paradigm Mastery Series.* St. Paul, MN: Star Thrower Distribution Corp.

Chopra, D. (1990). *Perfect Health.* New York: Harmony Books.

Clark, MJ. *Nursing in the Community.* (2nd ed.) Norwalk, CT: Appleton & Lange.

Federal Registry. (1995). 60(27), February 9.

Giger, J. & Davidhizar, R. (1995). *Transcultural Nursing: Assessment and Intervention.* (2nd ed.) St. Louis, MO: Mosby, p. 65.

Lagnado, L. (1996). Oxford to create alternative-medicine network. *The Wall Street Journal,* October 7.

Leininger, M. (1995). *Transcultural Nursing: Concepts, Theories, Research & Practices.* New York: McGraw-Hill.

Ornish, D. (1993). *Eat More, Weigh Less.* New York: HarperCollins.

Spector, R. (1996). *Guide to Heritage Assessment and Health Traditions.* Stamford, CT: Appleton & Lange, pp. 8–10.

6.

Application of Knowledge Base

The knowledge and insights you have acquired through your study of nursing concepts and practice and your experiences gained in the nursing specialties thus far are available to you whenever needed. The information in this chapter related to critical thinking skills and refining your assessment skills will continue to expand your knowledge base for practice in community based nursing.

APPLICATION OF THE NURSING PROCESS

The nursing process is the structure that directs your nursing practice. Each step of the nursing process is studied separately: assessment, diagnosis, planning, implementation, and evaluation. This approach allows you to become familiar with the characteristics of each step (Wilkinson, 1992). These steps appear isolated, yet in reality, they all flow together. Professional nurses move quickly from one step to another. In community based practice, the nurse often cares for a client over a period of time, which may result in application of various steps of the nursing process to different problems simultaneously.

A review of each step of the nursing process with examples of applications to community based practice is presented below (Wilkinson, 1992). Notice the more expanded focus of the nursing process in community based nursing when you compare it to hospital nursing.

Assessment

In the first step of the nursing process, you gather information, data, and facts from available sources. There may be a number of sources to consider. These sources can include the client, the family/caregiver, unlicensed personnel, referral information, the medical record, and other agencies and professionals that are involved in the client's care. This step is limited to data collection and can be accomplished through the following methods:

- Client assessment
- Family/caregiver assessment
- Community assessment
- Assessment of needed equipment
- Data gathering from caregivers
- Data gathering from multidisciplinary team

Client, family, and community assessments are discussed in detail later in the chapter.

Diagnosis

You use your critical thinking skills to synthesize the data you collect into a concise problem statement or a nursing diagnosis. The nursing diagnosis identifies the client's health status and links the actual or potential cause of that problem with the phrase "related to." An example is: High risk for altered parenting related to unrealistic expectation for infant.

Nursing diagnosis determines the direction the actual nursing care is to take. Nursing activities associated with the nursing diagnosis step include:

- Formulation of client diagnoses, including strengths
- Family diagnosis, including strengths
- Collaborating with client, family and others in prioritizing diagnoses

The North American Nursing Diagnosis Association (NANDA), which meets every two years, has created and is continually revising a list of nursing diagnoses. That list now consists of approximately 100 diagnoses. The Diagnosis Review Committee, one of eleven committees of this organization, updates the list by adding and deleting diag-

noses. Nurses can submit diagnoses to this committee for considera-
tion (NANDA, 1211 Locust Street, Philadelphia, PA 19107).

The use of NANDA-approved nursing diagnoses has traditionally
been most appropriate for hospital nursing because it focuses on reducing patient risks and vulnerabilities. In community based nursing,
the NANDA list is applicable to the specific problems of the client.
However, the identification of individual, family, and community
strengths, an assessment that is done routinely in community based
nursing, cannot be classified as a problem. In order to address this aspect, four **wellness diagnoses** have recently been added to the NANDA
list: (1) anticipatory grieving; (2) effective breast feeding; (3) family
coping; and (4) health-seeking behaviors. In time, more wellness la-
bels will be added (Stolte, 1996).

Be creative in your practice by developing diagnoses that accurately represent or describe positive aspects of your clients' lives. Community based nursing often involves aspects and/or problems of family life and the community when giving nursing care to a client. It is
important to include this relevant data in your nursing diagnosis.

Planning

Before proceeding into the planning step, it is important to note that
another step, **outcome identification**, precedes planning. The discussion surrounding this new addition has two sides. One side states that
outcome identification is already a part of or a precursor to planning.
The other side maintains that a separate step is needed to ensure outcome identification is incorporated into the nursing process. There is
a definite argument for its inclusion as critical paths or pathways and
other outcome criteria are used more and more in community settings and may be required for reimbursement of care. The development of outcome identification as a separate step of the nursing
process would support these changes.

Planning is the third step in the nursing process during which
you and the client set goals for working on the stated problems and
decide on the specific actions needed to reach the stated goals. The
factors involved in this step are as follows:

- Write goals in measurable terms.
- Classify goals as both short-term and long-term.
- Include the client and family/caregivers in teaching plans.
- Plan for your next scheduled appointment or visit.

Implementation

In implementation, the fourth step in the nursing process, the specific actions agreed upon in the planning step are actually carried out. These actions can be completed by the client, the caregiver, the nurse, or any other designated person. The actions and the outcomes are documented in the client's chart and communicated to other team members. These interventions consist of:

- Implementing the short- and long-term goals
- Teaching the client and family/caregivers
- Performing specific procedures
- Using appropriate community resources
- Collaborating with team members
- Delegating activities
- Documenting in reimbursable terms

Evaluation

Evaluation is the last step in the nursing process and the one in which you determine if the goals set in the planning step were achieved. Remember, evaluation is an ongoing process. For example, if you or the client decide that one of the actions in the planning step is not workable, it is replaced by another action. You are continuously evaluating each step and making necessary adjustments. The specific activities conducted during this step are:

- Assessing the level of the client's progress toward a goal
- Analyzing the effectiveness of the plan of care
- Revising the plan of care
- Evaluating outcomes

ASSESSMENT SKILLS

Most of the assessments you made in the hospital were related to the physical and mental status of the patient. In community based practice, these types of assessments are conducted with the client in the home or at the agency, with the family, and with the community. The combination of these three assessments gives you a comprehensive picture of the client and greatly influences your practice.

In the hospital, the patient is physically separated from his environment, which facilitates the performance of the necessary physical and mental assessments. There are few distractions. In community based nursing, beginning with your entry into the client's community and continuing into the home, the nurse is inundated with information about the client's environment, lifestyle, and interactions. The nurse must decide which information is relevant. The forms that the agency requires you to complete determine the client data, information, and facts that you will need to gather. Even if much of the information discussed below is not required for completing the forms, it will give you valuable insights that can assist you in your practice. Assessment of the community is followed by family assessment and client assessment. This is to remind you to consider the influence of each of these areas on the client's life even if you are not able to observe the community and family during a client appointment.

Community Assessment

This section is presented from the perspective of a home visit. If you are working with a client in an agency, you must remind yourself that the client lives in a community. You may drive to the community where the agency is located and where most of the clients who are seen at that agency reside. You can ask the client questions in order to obtain pertinent data about the impact of the client's environment on his life and on his medical condition.

As you live your life, you are continuously making assessments or noticing what is around you. In your practice, you will be fine-tuning your assessments in a specific, systematic way. Through your senses, a great deal is revealed about a community. In addition to what you see, are there smells? What is the feel about the place? A few of the questions you will be asking yourself are: "What are some of the potential strengths and liabilities of this community?" and "How is all of this related to my client?" The accompanying display presents areas to be evaluated during a community assessment.

If you work within the same community on a consistent basis, the community becomes very familiar to you. That familiarity is often accompanied by patterns of thinking that cause you to be on "automatic pilot" and as a result, you will not experience the community as you did initially. An example of this is the installation of a new stop sign in your immediate neighborhood that you literally do not see.

In the automatic mode, it is possible to miss the significance of the impact of the community on the client and family. An awareness of this

GENERAL OBSERVATIONS RELATED TO COMMUNITY ASSESSMENT

- **Type of Community**

    Urban: degree of congestion, traffic conditions
    Rural: degree of isolation
    Socioeconomic level
        Type of housing
    Industry
        Light (furniture, textiles, food stuffs, manufacturing)
        Heavy (steel, shipbuilding, mining, auto manufacturing)
    Is this the kind of community people move to or away from?

- **Activity within Community**

    Active
    Quiet
    Animal control
    Traffic patterns

- **General Condition of:**

    Roads
    Structures

- **Availability and Accessibility of**

    Grocery, hardware and other stores
    Gas stations
    Health care providers and facilities
    Places of worship
    Public Transportation
    Schools
    Restaurants
    Parks

response and the effort made to keep a focus on the client and what she may need can keep you open to what is in the routine environment.

Family Assessment

If you are making home visits during your community based nursing experience, then you will be making assessments related to the family. If the client is seen in an agency, you will not have the opportunity to do an assessment through your observations of that environment. However, it can still be helpful to go through this material so you will make the connection of the client to his family even though you may never meet the family.

PHYSICAL STRUCTURE OF THE HOME

- **Outside**
  - Describe the structure
  - Condition of outside area

- **Inside**
  - Adequacy and condition of furnishings
  - Telephone
    - Emergency numbers accessible
  - Environment
    - Orderly/cluttered
    - Temperature and ventilation
    - Lighting
    - Plumbing
    - Appliances
  - Safety
    - Bathroom and kitchen
    - Smoke detectors
    - Fire extinguishers
    - Stairs: well lit and uncluttered, handrails
    - Electrical
      - Cords and outlets
    - Other hazards

FAMILY STRUCTURE

Who lives in the household?
Ages
What is their relationship to each other?
Blood relatives or significant others
Extended family

FAMILY FUNCTION

- **Roles**

    Do family members work?
    Kind of work
    Office, laborer, etc.
    Educational level
    Literate?
    Hours members of the household are at home
    Are resources adequate?
    Sleep patterns of household members
    Who does the shopping, cooking, household chores?
    Who is the caregiver of the household?

- **Communication patterns and power**

    How are decisions made within family?
    How are conflicts resolved?
    How does the family cope with stress?
    Boundaries and rules
    How does family interact with their outside world?
    Friends, neighbors, church, and others
    Beliefs family holds about itself

It is a privilege to be invited into someone's home to assist them with their health needs. Our culture believes in the sanctity of the home; a place where people can be who they are in a self-determined way. In addition to assessing the problems, weaknesses, or vulnerabilities of a family, it is essential to assess the strengths or positive aspects as well. Getting in touch with these strengths can provide the force or resource for individuals and families to deal effectively with their problems or challenges.

In working in community based settings, you need to review your knowledge about family, including the developmental stages of families, family structure, and family functioning. The general information that can be gathered from the accompanying displays can be helpful to you in your nursing practice. The words "family" and "household" are used interchangeably.

Your agency may have specific assessment forms, such as safety of the home, that you will need to fill out. You may not be asked to assess many of the above categories. However, you can miss important, interrelated parts of the client's problem or resources if these areas are overlooked.

Family Function Related to the Client

Anything that has happened to the client with an illness, no matter what the diagnosis, has happened to the entire family. If the condition or illness is newly diagnosed, then the client and family members may still be adjusting and doing everything they can to maintain the family's equilibrium. Each person in the family and the family as a whole need to be assessed for where they are in the grieving process if the illness involves loss, whether it be a loss of function or impending loss of life.

The care of the ill client creates the need for adjustments in family members' daily lifestyles, such as family routines, schedules, priorities, finances, hopes, and dreams. Accurate assessments of the family need to include all of these areas and be expanded to include the family's coping skills, flexibility, and ability to learn about and assume responsibility for care. The answers to the following questions can provide much needed information.

- Who is able to assist with the client's care?
- Who is willing to assist?
- What are the family's beliefs about the client's illness?

Client Assessment

The individual assessment of the client is your primary focus. You are in the home because of a referral related to a specific client problem. The information you gathered about the community and family will begin to fall into place as you assess the client.

Community based agencies will require nurses to complete specific forms. In addition to payor and insurance forms, these usually include general client information, socioeconomic data, medical information, and data related to activities of daily living. Objective data is obtained by an initial complete physical examination and specific diagnostic and laboratory testing. If there are parts of the physical assessment that you feel less confident performing than others, you need to review the systems involved and have another professional assist you. Be continuously on the alert to update any of your assessment skills.

This individual assessment identifies the client's strengths and weaknesses and provides a baseline for later visits. Agencies that focus on mental health issues may require you to do a mental health assessment while others, like hospice, may need a spiritual assessment. The forms provided by the agency will determine which assessments are required and how comprehensive they need to be.

Medications, both prescription and nonprescription, need to be identified by name of medication, dosage, and frequency of administration. Again, an agency form is usually provided for recording this information. This assessment is done by asking the client to see his medications and comparing what the client is taking with the physician's orders. The more medications that are prescribed for each day, the greater the possibility of the client misunderstanding the purpose of the drugs and the times they are to be taken. It is a good idea to have the client or his caregiver tell you about each medication. In this way, any discrepancies of how much or when the client takes the medications become clear. You can also get an idea of his understanding about the actions of his medications.

CRITICAL THINKING SKILLS

The tendency with thinking, as with most things, is to think in habitual ways or in specific patterns. Critical thinking interrupts these patterns and causes us to question how we think, how we come to the conclusions we formulate, and how we solve problems.

Critical thinking makes the process of creative thinking possible. As you become aware of and enhance your critical thinking skills, you will ask questions about your practice, for example, how am I reasoning through this situation? In addition, you will be assessing your level of knowledge and the application of that knowledge.

As you read journal articles and books, it is important to continuously ask questions related to their validity in your nursing practice and in your life. As a culture, we tend to believe what is printed without much questioning. This is true in nursing, too. An example of this is the Patient's Bill of Rights initially developed by the American Hospital Association in 1973. As one reads this document, it looks comprehensive and valid. Questions one may raise are: "Who is to determine the rights of patients?" "Is it the place of the hospital, represented by their association, to decide what a patient's rights are?" "Wouldn't this be the same as men determining what women's rights should be or the young spelling out the rights of the aged population?" Perhaps rather than entitling the document "Patient's Bill of Rights," it needed to be labelled "The Hospital's Responsibilities to the Patient." We need to raise such questions to put things into perspective.

Tradition, or the way things have always been done, is another area for the application of critical thinking. The story is told about the young couple who were recently married. The wife is preparing a ham for dinner. She cut off both ends of the ham before putting it into the roasting pan. Her husband asked her why she did that. She responded: "My mother always did it." The husband, still not satisfied, wanted to know why. The young lady called her mother and asked her why she always cut the ends off the ham before putting it into the pan. The mother responded: "Grandma always did it." The mother called her mother and asked the question. The grandmother said: "Because it wouldn't fit in the pan."

In nursing, there are traditional ways of doing things that need to be questioned. An example is a nurse who is wheeling a patient face first into the elevator as someone held the "open door" button. Another nurse standing at the elevator said: "Turn her around!" The nurse turned the wheelchair around and backed the patient into the elevator. Later, the nurse asked herself two questions: "Why is it so important to back the patient in a wheelchair into the elevator? Is it so crucial that the patient face forward in the elevator?" The nurse who was criticized continued to wonder. Over time, she watched patients being wheeled into elevators, some wheeled in backwards and others forward. Then, one day the answer occurred to her. Years ago, when an elevator reached a floor, the place where the elevator and floor met were not always flush or in alignment. If you pushed the wheelchair with the patient facing forward into the elevator, you would not know if there was a drop of an inch or so which could cause injury to the patient. Today, because of technology, the elevator stops flush each time. If someone is pushing the button to hold the elevator open, the direction of the wheelchair really does not matter; the real danger no longer exists.

The application of scientific knowledge to your nursing practice in the community requires critical thinking. This can be true in the application of family developmental factors, interpersonal skills, and principles of sterile or clean technique. You may also observe the client improvising in a creative way which can stimulate your creative thinking.

Learning to be a critical thinker takes time; it is an attitude. It consists of continuously asking questions, questions about yourself and how you think, about your ideas, your beliefs, and how you do things. You become aware of how you think while you are thinking. Your inquisitive mind perserveres when questions arise. This process of inquiry encompasses your life, both personal and professional. It becomes part of who you are.

COMMUNITY INFORMATION

An accurate way to determine what an agency or institution values is to assess the information you are required to document in the client's record. With most agencies, the tendency is not to waste time doing things that are not required.

In most community based agencies, knowledge about the community, populations, and risk factors is not required and therefore this information is often ignored. Although collection of this knowledge may not be required, its availability can enhance your nursing practice. Many of your clients and their families may not fit into the categories of knowledge that you have learned and applied to the community. However, if this knowledge is appropriate to specific clients, it broadens your understanding and can lead to appropriate interventions. Gathering facts from the public health arena can help you to assist clients and their families to solve their problems. The public health concepts such as demographics and epidemiology can help you to identify valuable information about the community.

Demographics

The clients you are assigned to live within a specific geographic area. The people who live there are unique and make that community what it is. The community changes as people move in and out. An influx of people creates growth while stagnation or deterioration usually occurs as the population of a community declines.

As you become familiar with your area, there are many questions you will need to ask yourself. For example, what is the general age composition of the population in your area? Is it composed of many elderly people, young families, or a combination of both? This information can be gathered from census data.

The U.S. Bureau of the Census conducts a massive survey of the population of the country every ten years. The end-product of this study includes data about the country as a whole, individual states, counties, and census tracts. A census tract consists of 3,000 to 6,000 people. The data or statistics collected are separated into a broad spectrum of categories. These categories include: age, sex, race, ethnic background, and socioeconomic status. In addition to the census report, the U.S. Bureau of the Census also performs surveys on labor, crime, and housing. These surveys can be found in any public library (Swanson & Albrecht, 1993).

Becoming familiar with the available information for your area gives you an added perspective. For example, you will know if there are pockets of people that had previously been hidden from you, such as very elderly people living alone or an influx of people from another

 exercise 6–1

Locate the latest census report in your public library and study it. List the information for your area that you think can have an impact on the health of its people.

....

....

....

....

....

....

exercise 6–2

Suppose you discovered a pocket of very elderly people who live in your geographic area.

List the kinds of potential problems you might expect to find in the following areas:

Physical

....

....

....

....

....

Emotional

....

....

....

....

....

Social

....

....

....

....

....

Spiritual

....

....

....

....

....

Socioeconomic

....

....

....

....

....

Society

....

....

....

....

....

What impact would each of these categories have on an elderly person's health status?

....

....

....

....

....

What resources would need to be available in a community to assist with these needs?

....

....

....

....

....

....

country. This information can alert you to the potential health issues that may arise in your area and give you insight into possible solutions.

Statistics is the term used for data or information about a particular subject that is presented in the form of numbers. **Vital statistics** consist of data related to births, deaths, marriages, divorces and adoptions. Many states have added the number of abortions performed to the list of vital statistics. Health-related statistics, such as the number of cases of specific communicable diseases, are provided by the Centers for Disease Control. The local health department is a resource for these types of statistics for the community and state.

Epidemiology

Very simply, **epidemiology** is the science concerned with the study of disease and injury in populations. The major concerns of this science are how disease is distributed throughout a community and the causes of those diseases. In other words, the occurrence of disease and the determining factors that led to the diseases or injuries are studied. The focus is on a defined population rather than on the specific individuals.

Epidemiology originally emphasized the study of infectious diseases or epidemics. An **epidemic** is when the number of cases of a disease, condition, or injury exceeds what normally occurs or is expected.

Communicable diseases were the major cause of death in the world around the turn of the nineteenth century. These diseases declined in the industrialized world due to improvements in sanitation and the development of immunizations. Today we have "epidemics" of chronic diseases in the United States. Heart disease, diabetes, and cancer are noninfectious diseases that are of epidemic proportions.

In searching for the cause(s) of disease, epidemiologists study who is **at risk**, meaning the probability of a person developing a disease or health problem. To answer that question, epidemiologists need to know what are the "risk factors" involved. A **risk factor** is any condition or situation that increases the probability of developing an unfavorable condition or disease. The epidemiologist identifies risk factors for individuals and studies the rate at which new disease develops in a community.

The occurrence of disease is complex, and there are many factors that contribute to its development. The epidemiologic triangle is a model that seeks to explain the interaction of host, agent, and environment as it relates to the patterns of disease in a community (Figure 6–1). An assumption is made that deviations from health result from

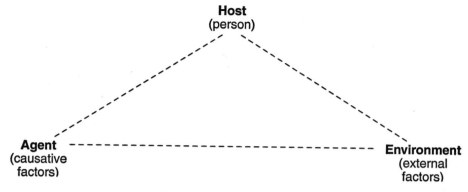

Figure 6–1. Epidemiologic triangle.

an imbalance among host, agent, and environment. These concepts are described below.

Host

The host is the person who is susceptible to a disease. Factors that influence susceptibility can be divided into two categories: (1) those factors over which the individual has no control, such as heredity, age, sex and race; and (2) those factors over which an individual has some degree of control, namely, lifestyle.

Agent

The agent is a causative factor that may be physical (heat, cold, friction), chemical (pesticides, chemicals, metals), or infectious (viruses, bacteria, parasites) in nature.

Environment

The environment consists of external factors that influence and contribute to the vulnerability of the host. Examples of these factors are the physical environment (climate, geography, temperature, rainfall, water and food supply, animal life, plants, insects), the psychosocial environment (social forces, resources and supports of the community, cultural influences, overcrowding) and the economic and working conditions (educational level, stress, access to health care, noise, poverty).

Epidemiologic Statistics

Public health data that you will encounter are often presented as rates. **Rates** are statistical measures that describe the proportion of in-

exercise 6–3

Using the epidemiologic triangle, list the factors that can contribute to a person developing tuberculosis.

Host:

....

....

....

....

....

Agent:

....

....

....

....

....

Environment:

....

....

....

....

....

dividuals with a specific disease or health problem in a population at risk within a unit of time. An example of this concept is the number of students who contracted the flu (individuals with a specific health problem) who are enrolled in X college (the population at risk) during the school year (unit of time).

To make rates easier to understand, a common base population of 1000 to 100,000 is used. Therefore, instead of using a fraction like

.000002, it is easier to compare the number of cases per 100,000 population in one city to another.

The statistical rates with which you want to be familiar are discussed below.

- *Mortality rate:* the number of reported deaths per 100,000 for midyear population (July 1) of a year.
- *Morbidity rate:* the rate that measures sickness or disease in a population.
- *Prevalence rate:* the rate of existing disease in a population at risk at a given time. An example would be the number of diabetics in a particular community at a given time.
- *Incidence rate:* the rate of new cases of a disease in a population at risk at a given time. This rate does not include the already existing cases. An example would be the number of newly diagnosed diabetics in the population at risk at a given time. The incidence rate gives you information about the risk of developing a disease.

A major focus of public health is the study of populations or aggregates of people rather than individuals. The knowledge gained from studying populations can be applied to individuals. An example of this was a British study that studied physicians who were smokers over a four and one-half year period. Studies that involve follow up of subjects over a period of time are known as prospective or cohort studies. It was known that people who smoked could develop lung cancer but the rate at which they developed it was not known. This study revealed that heavy smokers were 23.7 times more likely to develop lung cancer than nonsmokers (Swanson and Albrecht, 1993). Inferences are made from the results of studying a population or aggregate to individuals.

The Framingham Heart study, and other similar studies, have had a great impact on the development of preventive measures like exercising, not smoking, and decreasing serum cholesterol through diet. Smoking, high blood pressure, elevated cholesterol levels, and lack of exercise were found to be associated with heart disease after studying 5209 adults beginning in 1949 until their deaths (Stanhope and Lancaster, 1996).

The major uses of epidemiological studies include: (1) finding the causes of disease; (2) applying the results of the study of a specific population group to individuals; (3) isolating risk factors for individuals; (4) determining the rate at which new disease develops in a community by comparing rates with other communities; and (5) using this information as evidence for deciding which health services are needed in a community.

To reiterate, you will not be required to collect or use this information in most community based agencies. However, it can give you many insights into the situations you are confronted with in the community and lead to excellence in your nursing practice.

REPORTABLE SITUATIONS OR CONDITIONS

The reporting of certain situations and conditions by health care professionals is mandatory by law. For example, vital statistics (births, deaths, marriages, and divorces) must be recorded and the records maintained in every state. In addition, most states require the reporting of abortions and neonatal deaths. Certain disorders or diseases, abuse, and unlocked loaded weapons are also subject to reporting and are discussed in detail below.

Reportable Diseases

Communicable diseases must be reported in order to protect the public. The list of reportable diseases in each state may vary, so again, it is important to familiarize yourself with the list of reportable diseases for the state in which you practice. For example, sexually transmitted diseases, cancer, and seizure disorders can be among the disorders or illnesses for which particular states require notification.

If you become aware of certain facts that cause you to question whether or not a client or family member has a reportable disease, follow-up is necessary. Check with your supervisor and/or the physician about the appropriate procedures involved with the reporting and management of these conditions.

Abuse

If you suspect or see evidence of abuse of a child, an elderly person, or anyone who is incapable of acting on his or her own behalf, you are required to report it. Abuse may be either in the form of medical, physical, or emotional neglect, or mental, physical, or sexual assault.

It was not until 1966 that all 50 states had laws for reporting suspected child abuse (Spradley & Allender, 1996). These laws continue to be refined. For example, in one state, a telephone call to Social Services about alleged child abuse is sufficient to initiate a process of follow-up by professionals. In another state, a written report about suspected abuse must be submitted within a certain length of time. The nurse who works in the community may be the only person who has the necessary information to file these types of reports with the appropriate agency. Therefore, it is essential that you know the laws related to abuse in your state. This cannot be stressed enough. You must report only the required information to the proper governmental agency. The nurse may be liable for reporting more than the required information or notifying the wrong agency. Nurses are more liable if they fail to report abuse than if they report only the required information to the proper agency (Guido, 1997). Know the policies and procedures relating to the reporting of suspected abuse established by your agency and work with your direct supervisor before taking action.

Weapons

The purchasing and possession of firearms by law abiding citizens in our country is a very controversial issue. Laws regarding weapons vary from state to state, so it is imperative that you know the laws in your area on gun control. The community based nurse is concerned with safety issues associated with gun possession.

Some people feel unsafe where they live and may keep a loaded weapon within reach for safety. If children live in the house or visit, possessing a loaded gun that they can potentially have access to can be lethal to them. There are various types of locks one can purchase to safeguard weapons. The argument expressed by some people against a lock is that the weapon is not ready to be discharged as needed. It is important to discuss the risk with family members, particularly children, of having an unlocked, loaded gun at home.

In your practice in the community, you can teach the client or family about safety measures related to a weapon: keeping the weapon locked up, keeping the gun and the ammunition locked up separately, and teaching children and other family members about firearms safety.

Some states have concealed weapon laws. These laws mean that citizens who meet the requirements may carry a concealed weapon. Even so, it is against the law to bring a weapon into designated buildings and areas. You need to know your agency's policies and procedures related to these issues so that, if a client is violating the law, you will know how to proceed.

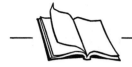

CHAPTER HIGHLIGHTS

1. Application of the nursing process in community based nursing includes the family and the community in addition to the client.

2. Assessment skills used in community based settings are broadened from the client to include the family and the community. Assessments from these three combined areas provide data, information, and facts that assist you in your community based nursing practice.

3. Refinement of your critical thinking skills encourages you to raise questions and creatively solve problems.

4. The application of public health concepts such as demographics and epidemiology can provide insights into community based nursing practice.

5. The laws for reporting communicable disease, abuse, and unsecured weapons vary from state to state and nurses in community based practice are required to be familiar with the provisions for notification and follow-up.

REFERENCES

Guido, G.W. (1997) *Legal Issues in Nursing.* (2nd ed). Stamford, CT: Appleton & Lange.

Spradley, B. & Allender, J. A. (1996). *Community Health Nursing.* (4th ed.) New York: Lippincott.

Stanhope, M. & Lancaster, J. (1996). *Community Health Nursing.* (4th ed.) St. Louis, MO: Mosby.

Stolte, K.M. (1996). *Wellness Nursing Diagnosis for Health Promotion.* Philadelphia: Lippincott.

Swanson, J.M. & Albrecht, M. (1993). *Community Health Nursing.* Philadelphia: W.B. Saunders.

Wilkinson, J. (1992). *Nursing Practice in Action: A Critical Thinking Approach.* New York: Addison-Wesley Nursing.

7.

Client Teaching

Teaching is a core function of the nurse who practices community based nursing. The more adept you are at teaching, the more you are able to help people help themselves. It is an art and a skill to assess and evaluate each client's learning needs and to mold your knowledge of teaching to the situation at hand. As you refine your teaching skills, your practice in community based settings will become more rewarding.

Before beginning relationships with clients, it is essential to reflect on the fact that these people had been living their lives as usual just a short time ago. Because of illness or disability, these clients were then thrust into an unknown system that is outside their paradigms. They were diagnosed with a disorder that perhaps can be cured or which may lead to a chronic condition for the rest of their lives. Their bodies were invaded and many were left with gaping wounds that may have drains protruding from them, sutures still in place, and dressings that need changing on a regular basis. With all of these changes, their attention span may now be shorter. These clients also need medications for pain and other symptoms. They are then sent home with paraphernalia they do not quite understand and wonder how they will manage at home with unskilled helpers—namely family members or significant others—and if their lives will ever be the same.

The nurse is often the first person to visit the client at home after he has been discharged from the hospital and has experienced the scenario described above. The quicker you are able to assess the knowledge level of the client and family the sooner you will be able to facilitate their independence. The manner in which the client and primary caregivers are able to perform necessary procedures and make supporting life-style changes can make the difference in the level of functioning the client is able to achieve.

Below is a review of the general principles of teaching and learning that you have previously learned and an application of these principles to the client in community based settings. These principles support learning. We separate these two intertwined sets of principles to be able to examine them closely just as we study the steps of the nursing process independently. As with the nursing process, you are aware that the elements of the teaching and learning process are closely related and are continuously evaluated. The principles of teaching are usually assigned to the nurse while the principles of learning are assigned to the client/family.

PRINCIPLES OF TEACHING AND LEARNING

Principles of teaching and learning provide a foundation for your teaching. Knowing what supports both teaching and learning can offer you insights into how to assist the client and family with what they need to learn.

Nursing Focus: Teaching

The following principles of teaching, personal philosophy, planning, development of teaching skills, rapport, communication, relevancy of information, amount of information, use of affective methods, and environment are discussed below.

Personal Philosophy
The beliefs the nurse has about the client, the family, and the disease or situation are subtly communicated. If you believe that something can be accomplished, then you will use all of your resources to that end. If, on the other hand, you do not believe something is possible, you will restrict your efforts and goals. Nursing students tend to believe that anything is possible and because of those beliefs they are often able to help clients conduct their lives in a more healthy manner in ways that staff nurses are unable to accomplish. It is important to remain open to others' ideas and beliefs and give people the benefit of the doubt.

Planning

In community based practice, every visit counts, so it is important to develop a plan of how you will teach the information that the client/family needs to learn at a particular time. This plan is specific to the client, reflects client input, and depends on your creativity to devise ways to simplify and clarify what the situation requires.

Development of Teaching Skills

As you begin your community based practice, you may feel that you are not an effective teacher. This feeling is perfectly acceptable. Self-evaluation of your skills is important and can lead to assessment of areas that need to be strengthened. If you find that you have problems teaching about a specific condition, learn as much as you can about the subject because a solid knowledge base will give you confidence and help you concentrate on ways in which you will communicate the subject matter to the client and family. Observe how your preceptor or peers approach a particular aspect of teaching and incorporate relevant elements into your teaching. Practice will give you confidence.

Rapport

Rapport is present when the relationship between the client and the nurse is in harmony and accord. To accept and appreciate people just as you find them is the basis for rapport. Your caring is clearly communicated through non-verbal behavior. When you are present, open, and listening intently, the client experiences acceptance. To be present means not thinking about what you have yet to accomplish throughout the day or anything else. After rapport is initially established, the nurse and the client must continuously work together to maintain that rapport because words, actions, attitudes, and beliefs can either strengthen or weaken this relationship.

Communication

The ability to communicate is directly related to the level of rapport you are able to establish. If the client trusts you, she will feel free to ask questions. Honesty on the part of both the nurse and the client/family leads to open communication and the freedom to discuss health-related issues without the fear of being judged or criticized. At times, if communication feels strained between you and the client, it is a good idea to gently investigate this issue with the client, because it may be related to how the client is feeling in general or it may be about something that was said or done.

Relevancy of Information

If the information you are teaching challenges the client/family within their limits and makes sense to them, their attention is more likely to be held and compliance with suggested changes is enhanced. If it has meaning for them, then the information is valued. Determine the point where the client is in her response to her situation and then gently move with her from that point in the direction of agreed upon goals.

The nurse can determine if information is relevant by paying attention to the amount of interest the client shows in the subject, the number and kinds of questions asked by the client, and the degree of willing participation and follow through. You may inadvertently be using terminology that the client is unable to understand. You may need to use visuals. As you interact with the client, it is acceptable to ask about the problems you perceive in the communication of the message and then change your plan accordingly.

Amount of Information

When a significant amount of information must be given to a newly diagnosed client, the tendency is to tell all you know about the condition. This approach can overwhelm or exhaust the client which leads to limited absorption of material. To avoid this situation, make a list of what you want the client to learn and then prioritize the list, starting with what is crucial for survival. Decide what you plan to cover during each visit and gradually communicate the relevant information to the client. Check periodically with the client to determine if he or she is at the point at which no additional information can be understood.

Use of Affective Methods

Affective methods are those that influence the client's emotions or feelings. There are times when appealing to the client's emotions, feelings, attitudes, and beliefs is a very useful teaching method. We are not talking about causing fear in someone. Fear usually captures a person's attention; however, the resulting changes often last only for a short time. Thus, fear as a motivator is basically ineffective. The client is seldom able to shift a major belief and permanently change a behavior as the result of fear. In addition, fear can undermine trust and destroy rapport; the cost to your relationship can be great. Gently nudging the client by stimulating positive feelings and attitudes within him is much more effective.

Environment

In a formal setting, such as a classroom, the teacher is responsible for the environment. In the client's home, the client creates the environment. However, you can make suggestions that support a learning environment within the home setting. For example, if the television or radio is so loud as to make it difficult to hear, you may state to the client that you have important information to give him and ask him if it would be acceptable to lower the volume for a few minutes. Make sure that the client and the environment are as comfortable as possible so that nothing interferes with the communication of information.

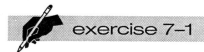

exercise 7-1

This exercise applies the principles in the section entitled "Nursing Focus: Teaching."

A young woman in her twenties lived in an abusive situation. She admitted herself and her three interracial children (ages 7, 9, and 10) into a Battered Womens' Shelter. A couple of years later, she died of AIDS.

The young woman's 52-year-old divorced mother has had custody of her three grandchildren since her daughter's death about a year ago. They live in public housing and are supported by public assistance. There are no relatives or close friends living in the vicinity. The three children attend public school while the grandmother stays at home. She freely talks about her daughter's "horrible" death and how many of the caregivers were unkind to her daughter when she became blind and was unable to help herself.

The grandmother is 5'6" tall and weighs approximately 170 pounds. Her blood pressure is taken as a screening measure on the first visit and the reading is 158/90. She states that she feels fine and offers no physical complaints. She has not seen a doctor in more than 20 years and states that as long as she feels good, she doesn't need to go to a doctor. "If I live my life correctly, God will take care of me." She often refers to her open Bible during the visit.

1. Could the concept of cultural imposition (see Chapter 5) become an issue in this case? In what way(s)?

   ....

   ....

   ....

2. What beliefs does this grandmother hold?

   ....

   ....

   ....

3. Apply the following principles of teaching to this case. How could each of them influence the direction that future visits take?
   a. Personal philosophy of the nurse

   ....

   ....

   ....

   ....

   ....

   b. Rapport

   ....

   ....

   ....

   ....

   ....

   c. Communication

   ....

   ....

   ....

   ....

   ....

   d. Relevance of information

   ....

   ....

....

....

e. Use of affective methods

....

....

....

....

4. From a focus of primary and secondary prevention, what would you ideally like to accomplish with this family? How would it be possible to accomplish these goals? Be creative.
   a. Primary prevention

....

....

....

....

   b. Secondary prevention

....

....

....

....

Client Focus: Learning

Principles such as domains of learning, learning styles, physical and mental readiness, perception, responsibility for learning, impact of emotions, active participation, imitation, repetition, and experiencing satisfaction greatly affect the client's ability to learn. Your awareness of these concepts as you are teaching can facilitate the process.

Domains of Learning

Learning is both cognitive and affective. Effective learning takes place when both of these domains are activated. To illustrate, when you consider the goals that you are in the process of achieving, there is both the thinking (cognitive) and the feeling or attitude (affective) parts to the process.

In the thinking part, you decide what it is you are able to accomplish and the facts about the goal. Your feelings or attitudes give momentum to the process. The combination of thinking and feeling creates a very powerful force that moves you in the direction you desire. In teaching a client, plan strategies that include facts as well as those that stimulate positive feelings.

Learning Styles

Learning styles are classified as being either visual, auditory or kinesthetic. Each person has a dominant style and is more or less able to change to a less dominant style. Most people are visual, which means they learn more quickly and easily by observing something or looking at pictures. The person who possesses an auditory learning style learns through hearing or listening. Kinesthetic learning occurs through touching or literally performing an action. In your teaching, because you do not know the client's dominant learning style, you need to engage as many of the senses as possible to enhance learning. An example of incorporating the various learning styles is illustrated below.

As the nurse was listening to a client describe what he was experiencing, she made note of the fact that he focused on the various parts involved in his condition and his perception of how they functioned. She asked what type of work he did. Learning that he was a mechanic provided her with a focus of how to present what he needed to know in a way that he could easily grasp.

Physical and Mental Readiness

It is important to assess the physical impairments that a client has that may affect his ability to learn. Many diseases cause loss of function. Your knowledge of the effects of disease on the body alerts you to potential physiologic changes in hearing, vision, neurologic, and/or perceptual functioning. In addition, mental readiness can be affected by these physical changes. The client may still be in the process of adjusting to dramatic shifts in his body and, in turn, in his life. An awareness of what the client is experiencing determines how you will proceed in your teaching.

Knowledge of growth and development principles helps you to determine the maturational aspects of the client that need to be taken into account. The educational level of the client influences how and in what form you present material. For instance, a picture may be more effective in communicating information than writing down words that the client may have difficulty understanding.

Everyone has a time of day when they function best. Usually, people who function best in the morning wake up cheerful, alert, and ready to participate in activities. People who function best in the evening may take time to wake up in the morning and need quiet until they are fully awake. Peak time for learning is the time of day when one can easily concentrate and is alert and receptive. If at all possible, schedule visits during or close to that time of day.

When teaching people who are sick or debilitated, the energy level of the person must be considered. Usually, the sicker the person, the greater the energy depletion and the smaller the energy reserve. Caution must be used to not further deplete the client's energy by prolonging the visit, asking the client to do too much at once, or covering too much material in one visit.

Perception

How one perceives a situation greatly influences learning. An example is a client with tuberculosis who would not keep her appointments at the clinic. The chart documented the efforts taken to encourage the client to keep an appointment. A new nurse assigned to the client asked her to describe her understanding of this situation. The client stated that she believed that if her TB was not cured, she would be admitted into a sanatorium and separated from her 10 year-old daughter. She said she would not be able to handle such a long-term separation. The nurse explained that if the client followed the medical regimen, it would facilitate her recovery and that keeping her appointments at the clinic would not lead to admission to a sanatorium. As a result of this information, the client's perception of the situation changed and she followed through on both the visits to the clinic and the course of treatment. The nurse listened intently, heard the client's beliefs, and was able to present knowledge that both appealed to the client's feelings and matched the presenting beliefs. This response made it possible for the client to shift her perspective and easily do what was necessary to enhance her state of health.

Responsibility for Learning

In some situations, the nurse can conduct appropriate teaching and yet the client and/or family may decide not to participate or to learn anything. The nurse may make many changes in teaching strategies in response to this behavior, but achieve few results. This situation can be difficult for the nurse to accept because she wants the best for her clients and their families. The nurse may also blame herself. It is important to remember that, whatever the reasons may be for the client not learning, it is a choice. As long as you have done everything that you are able to do and have fulfilled your responsibilities as a teacher, you can free yourself of assuming responsibility for the client's/family's learning.

Impact of Emotions

If a client has just been given a life-threatening diagnosis, is in pain, feels that her situation is hopeless, or is in any strong emotional state, you can expect that her perceptions about her condition may be distorted. She may not be able to hear what you are saying, the information may not be absorbed, or there may be selective hearing. It is important to assess this aspect before you begin teaching so that you can choose appropriate methods that may help you in communicating with this client.

Active Participation

The more involved the client is in the process of caring for herself, the more receptive she is likely to be to new learning. Again, listen for her beliefs about her situation. Many times, the client believes she can accomplish whatever is at hand and she wants to be involved in the effort to maximize her health. These clients are a joy to work with because the process flows easily. The challenge comes into play when the client has no interest in participating. In this type of relationship, you need to explore the client's feelings about this response to learning. Assisting the client in turning this situation around creates satisfaction within the nurse.

Imitation

It is easier to do something after you have watched someone else do it because you are able to imitate what you have seen. Whatever you need to teach, have the person(s) present who are responsible for performing the procedure. While observing the steps of the process, they can ask questions and gain confidence about doing it themselves.

Repetition

The more times a person is able to perform something, the easier it is to do. The repetition increases skill and builds self-confidence. The more self-confidence the person has, the easier it is to proceed. As an example, consider the new diabetic to whom you are teaching self-administration of insulin. The client observes you prepare and administer the insulin while you give verbal instructions. The next time, the client is given the opportunity to prepare and self-administer the insulin. This skill becomes easier for the client with practice. Repetition in performance and redundancy in giving directions strengthens learning by clarifying how various steps are to be done and the correct sequence of those steps.

Experiencing Satisfaction in Learning

Success in learning is a source of satisfaction. When the client is able to master one aspect of caring for himself, this creates self-confidence and the impetus to learn more. Positive reinforcement and support encourages the client and family and contributes to feelings of accomplishment. These experiences produce positive outcomes that lead to independence in care.

ASSESSMENT OF CLIENT TEACHING NEEDS

Your assessment begins with the referral for a visit. Read the referral carefully to learn as much information as possible. If you have any questions about the client's diagnosis, review your anatomy and physiology book to assess the systems affected by the condition. Check a nursing skills procedure book to review a procedure that you may not have performed recently.

Research the medications that have been prescribed for the client in the *Physician's Desk Reference* (PDR). Find a pharmacy that provides a print-out of information about the medications and file them in a notebook in alphabetical order. Many of the same medications are prescribed for different clients with the same diagnosis. Then, at any given point, you are able to open your book to the medication and quickly review the actions, food–drug interactions, side effects, and other special directions.

Teaching and the Initial Home Visit

On your way to the home for the initial visit, conduct general assessments related to safety, the community, and the home. (See Chapter 6 for discussion about these assessments.) The continuous assessments you make about aspects related to the client provide you with valuable data to include in planning, implementing, and evaluating your nursing care.

As you communicate with the client, family, or significant others and establish rapport, you are continuously making assessments of the client and family in the following areas:

- Ability to listen
- Level of comprehension
- Educational level
- Cultural influences
- Availability of resources
- The role of significant others
- Understanding of the diagnosis
- The meaning of diagnosis to the client/family

Before you begin teaching, you need to determine the client's level of understanding about his condition or disease and what it means to him. Assess whether the client has prior knowledge of or experience with the subject area to be taught. You want to move from the familiar to the unfamiliar and the simple to the complex.

If the client makes a statement that indicates a misunderstanding about his condition or disease, explore this situation. Listen to every word the client says because the beliefs that the client holds are expressed in these statements. This exchange of information helps you to know if the possibility of change in perspective is a matter of additional knowledge or if the reason for refusal of change is based on strongly held beliefs, like religious beliefs. Once you are able to determine this, then you will know where to begin your teaching and you may also be able to suggest an alternative plan that can incorporate the client's beliefs and thus be more acceptable to the client.

Remember, the words that you choose and the tone and volume of your voice are tools that you need to refine in order to be an effective teacher. How you use these tools can make the difference in whether or not the client complies with the treatment regime. For example, if you need to communicate something of special importance, you can move closer to the client by leaning forward, establish direct eye contact (if the client's culture permits this action), and speak slowly using a soft voice. This approach is very different from proceeding in a normal voice at a normal pace.

As your assessment continues, you want to consider any social factors that you think may influence learning. Are there cultural influences that may have an impact on learning? Is there a language barrier? If so, focus on presenting one idea at a time using simple sentence structures and examples that are concrete rather than conceptual (Price & Cordell, 1994).

You will be continuously assessing and evaluating during the visit. This serves two purposes. First, it allows you to become acquainted with the client and her situation, establish rapport and refrain from the tendency to label or judge situations. You now have vital information as to what the client needs to learn and how to proceed in communicating that knowledge. The other purpose is to help the client get to know you, learn that you care about and accept her, and that the two of you will be working together for the purpose of improving her situation.

Pay particular attention to any feelings or attitudes within you that are stimulated during this visit. Are they positive or negative? What beliefs do you hold about the client/family situation?

Awareness of the literacy of the client is an important aspect of this process. We tend to assume that everyone can read and write. However, it is estimated that about 20% of adults in our country are functionally illiterate (Doak, Doak, & Root, 1996). Illiterate clients are not likely to admit this problem to you because of embarrassment. Clues that may point to deficiencies in reading and writing skills are the absence of books, newspapers, magazines, pens or pencils within the environment, or if the client signs a document with an "X."

A positive aspect about this situation is that it reminds you that this issue of literacy does not mean that the client is unable to learn. Instead you need to adjust your teaching strategies in order to establish an effective relationship. This modification includes the level of information and terminology used to communicate it. The client's attention span may be short. Keep it simple. Use visuals, and as you do with any client, explain something several different ways, and use different examples. Move from the simple to the complex and be aware of the pace at which material is being assimilated.

Client Readiness to Learn

It is a great advantage if the client is ready to learn. Readiness and motivation are intertwined. As you interact with the client and family, in addition to listening for the expression of beliefs, you want to be alert to hints and other evidence that the client is prepared to learn. For instance, is there a general engagement or interest in your visit? Does the client demonstrate an eagerness to know what he already has experienced or is presently experiencing? Does the client or family ask questions? A client or caregiver may directly ask about how to do something related to his care.

Another clue of readiness to learn is the client describing to you how someone he knows performed a specific action. Interest is evident if the client or family member reposition themselves in order to fully observe whatever you are doing.

You want to make sure that you provide periods of silence during your teaching. This technique gives the client time to process what is being communicated, synthesize information, and formulate questions. The silence may be needed to just "be" at that moment.

Client/Family Involvement

As you plan your teaching strategies, you need to involve the client, family, or significant others who will be participating in the client's care. Share your priorities with them. If you can give the client various choices as to the specific content that needs to be taught, the client can experience a degree of control over the schedule. Discuss the plan of care with the client and family.

Share your expectations of the relationship with the client. For example, you may state that, during the next visit, you will guide the client as she prepares and administers insulin to herself and suggest that she review the written instructions. This approach can take the mystery, fear, or uncertainty out of what is going to happen next. It also gives the client and family members a chance to clarify their concerns.

Leave written instructions as needed. As necessary, certain instructions can be presented in the form of pictures which is an effective way to explain procedures.

FEEDBACK

When you or the client give feedback about information exchanged, you are communicating your perspectives. Feedback is a judgment that can either be positive or negative. Constructive feedback encourages confidence and helps the person to understand the level of success in meeting expectations. Negative feedback, without positive comments, can undermine self-confidence and cause discouragement. When a procedure is being performed incorrectly, it is important to make the client aware of mistakes. How this feedback is presented can determine if the client perceives it as negative or positive.

The provision of feedback is an important responsibility of the nurse as teacher. Below is a list of general guidelines for you to follow in giving feedback to the client (Rankin & Stallings, 1996).

- Give feedback as soon as possible, such as immediately after performing a procedure.

- Give positive aspects or strengths of performance first, then, discuss weaknesses or what needs to be done differently.
- Focus on the behavior rather than the person.
- Be aware of the amount of information you are giving and avoid, overloading the client with details.
- Orient your comments to the present.

EVALUATION OF TEACHING

As you continuously evaluate your teaching, you create a flow of the process of teaching and learning rather than definite steps. Your evaluation of your strategies leads to reassessment and modification of your techniques. Changes in goals and teaching strategies are the result of evaluations made by you and/or others and are made as the need for change is presented.

DOCUMENTATION

You need to document any client teaching that you conduct with the client, family, and/or caregiver. Community based agencies have guidelines for documenting your teaching that need to be followed. These guidelines are based on Medicare, Medicaid, and insurance company standards that determine reimbursement.

Your entry needs to include the content of your teaching, the person to whom the teaching was primarily directed, and anyone else who was observing the process. If you gave a demonstration, state the actions demonstrated, the person who performed a return demonstration, and the provision of an opportunity to ask questions. Include some of the questions asked by the client in your entry if there was anything out of the ordinary or that raised questions in your mind. Document any instructions you gave to the client, family, and/or caregiver of what they are to do if they encounter a problem in providing care.

Reimbursement and Client Teaching

Many home care agencies are structured on the managed care model. Managed care consists of providing the best care possible while controlling unnecessary access to the agency's resources. Under this system, the nurse is informed of the number of home visits that are allotted to teach a patient with a certain diagnosis. For example, you may have five home visits to teach a newly diagnosed diabetic. The teaching includes an understanding of the disease, insulin administration, signs and symptoms of hyperglycemia and hypoglycemia, diet, foot care, and living with the disease. On the initial visit, let the client and family know how many visits you will be making and for what purpose. This information places a value on the visits so that time is not occupied with visitors, television programs, or other distractions.

The other type of reimbursement structure is the open-ended payment structure. The number of visits in which the teaching is conducted will be flexible so the nurse is able to adjust the number of visits to the needs of the client. For example, if a client has low literacy skills and needs additional visits to master the stated learning objectives, an increase in the number of visits is possible. The advantages to this reimbursement structure includes pacing the learning to the client rather than to the disease and being confident that the client has adequate time to accomplish what is needed. The disadvantage is that the nurse may take more time than is needed, thus costing the agency more money.

MEDICARE REQUIREMENTS FOR TEACHING

Medicare has specific requirements related to reimbursement and non-reimbursement of teaching. The following is a summary of both (Hunt & Zurek, 1997).

Reimbursable teaching is:

- Teaching that is conducted to manage the prescribed treatment.
- Teaching that is necessary and reasonable; that is, the teaching is related to the client's functional loss or to the illness or injury.

In the initial teaching, you determine the number of visits that are necessary and reasonable by the complexity of what you need to teach and the learner's ability. In subsequent teaching, you determine the number of necessary and reasonable visits by how much was retained by the client and what you anticipate the learning progress to be.

Generally, non-reimbursement for teaching is applicable if:
- The client, family, or caregiver is unable to learn.
- There is an absence of documentation as to the reason learning did not occur.

 exercise 7–2

At what level(s) of prevention is one teaching when the directions refer to the client's functional loss or to her illness or injury?

....

....

....

....

....

Explain.

....

....

....

....

....

What changes, if any, do you think need to be made in the Medicare regulations for reimbursement of teaching?

....

....

....

....

....

....

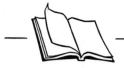

CHAPTER HIGHLIGHTS

1. Teaching is a major role of the community based nurse.

2. Principles of teaching relate to the function of the nurse, and include personal philosophy, planning, development of teaching skills, rapport, communication, relevancy of information, amount of information, use of affective methods, and environment.

3. Principles of learning relate to the client/caregiver and include domains of learning, learning styles, physical and mental readiness, perception, responsibility for learning, impact of emotions, active participation, imitation, repetition, and experiencing satisfaction.

4. A thorough assessment of teaching needs leads to an accurate plan of care, workable teaching strategies, and appropriate reimbursement.

5. Positive and constructive feedback gives the client/caregiver an evaluation of performance.

6. Evaluation of teaching can lead to a reordering of priorities, new strategies, and more effective outcomes.

7. Documentation of teaching must be done according to agency guidelines.

8. Medicare requirements for teaching determine reimbursement eligibility and impact the practice of nursing.

REFERENCES

Doak, C., Doak, L. and Root, J. (1996). *Teaching Patients with Low Literacy Skills.* (2nd ed.) Philadelphia: J.B. Lippincott Co., p. 3.

Hunt, R. and Zurek, E. (1997). *Introduction to Community Based Nursing.* Philadelphia: J.B. Lippincott Co., p. 200.

Price, J. and Cordell, B. (1994). Cultural diversity and patient teaching. *Journal of Continuing Education in Nursing* 25:4.

Rankin, S. and Stallings, K. (1996). *Patient Education: Issues, Principles, Practices.* (3rd ed.) Philadelphia: J.B. Lippincott Co., pp. 230–231

IV.

....

PRACTICE SETTINGS IN COMMUNITY BASED NURSING

....

8.

Home Visiting

The general information covered thus far applies to nursing practice in all types of community based settings: clinics, offices, schools, centers, and in the home. This chapter focuses on aspects of nursing practice specifically related to the care of clients in their homes. This information is also valuable to those nurses who make infrequent home visits. The nurses who make home visits on a consistent basis are usually employed by home care agencies and hospice.

Confidentiality, preparing for the initial home visit, planning your day, the initial visit, availability of equipment and supplies, infection control standards, and documentation and recordkeeping are particularly relevant to the delivery of nursing care in the home and are discussed below.

PREPARING FOR THE INITIAL HOME VISIT

As discussed in Chapter 1, the nurse is a guest in the client's home. The anticipation of going into a stranger's home to assist with nursing care can be frightening and nurses may experience a range of fears.

The accompanying display provides guidelines for your physical safety. Following these guidelines can help you avoid many potential problems.

The most basic principle is that your **personal safety comes first**. Trust your intuition or "gut feeling." For example, a student, who was completing some paperwork in her car outside a client's house after a

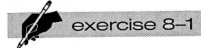 exercise 8–1

In your clinical group, each student is to list the fears he or she feels about going to a stranger's home to practice nursing.

The lists are collected and read by one person. Each fear is discussed by the group.

....

....

....

....

....

visit, looked up and saw a person walking in her direction who frightened her. She double checked her locked car doors and then drove off. The student's intuition was speaking loudly to her.

It is wise and prudent to pay attention to that feeling. Similarly, if a client has visitors and something does not feel right, ask the client for an appropriate time for you to return. The bottom line is: **never ignore your intuition.**

Another concern with conducting home visits is getting lost. Always carry a current local map. If a map is not provided by the agency, obtain one from the Chamber of Commerce or other agency that distribute maps. Make sure the map includes the circumference of the area in which you expect to be traveling. You will have the addresses of the clients you are to visit before you leave the office. The first step is to find the street on the map and decide on the route to be taken. Agency staff are a great resource. If still unsure of the directions, when you call the client to negotiate a time for your visit, ask for directions. By the time you leave for the visit, you will have a clear picture of where you will be going.

CONFIDENTIALITY

In the practice of home visiting, you take confidential information pertaining to your clients with you. This data is moved from your car, to the

SAFETY GUIDELINES FOR HOME VISITING

- Keep your car doors locked at all times.
- Put any personal items in the trunk before leaving for home visits.
- Make certain you have an adequate amount of fuel in your car. When you are between visits, you should not have to be concerned about whether or not you are going to run out of gas and thus have to worry about finding a gas station.
- Keep your car in good condition so it functions effectively and safely.
- Carry a cellular phone at all times or have change to make a phone call.
- If possible, park in well-lit areas and in a place where you are not alone in dimly lighted areas.
- Be aware of the surroundings at all times.
- Remember, these are considerations that apply to everyday living, not just your work life.

house, within the house, and back to your car. Therefore, it is important to develop a system to ensure effective organization of and easy access to this information. You need to remember that, during your visit, it is possible for someone in the home, such as a neighbor, to peruse your paperwork while you are busy with the client in another room. In addition, you can understand why locking your car each time you leave it is imperative. Even though you lock your car, however, it is possible for it to be stolen, so you need to think carefully about what you leave in the car.

Organization of Equipment and Supplies

Accessibility to the equipment and supplies needed in your community based nursing practice takes thought, planning, and organization. In the hospital, the nurse does not have to give much attention to what she will need to deliver care. Going to another department to get an item that is short stocked on the unit is very often viewed as an an-

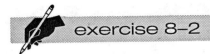

exercise 8-2

Take a moment now and recall an incident when you were
very frightened.
    Where in your body did you get the message?

....

....

....

....

....

....

....

noyance. But think for a moment about the consequences of not having what you need when you are making a visit 15 or more miles from
the agency. In fact, no matter how organized your supplies are, there
will be times when it is impossible to predict your needs or anticipate
items not present in the home. During those times, you and the
client/caregiver may need to develop a creative plan through which
certain supplies can be improvised from standard items in the home.
Therefore, using a system through which you are continuously aware
of your inventory is more than a want; it is a necessity.
    The supply room of home care and hospice agencies is a major
area of concern because of the cost of the equipment and supplies
contained in it. Some agencies exercise very tight controls over the
items that leave that room and have established a documentation trail
leading to the use of each item. Other agencies are more lenient
about the use of supplies. Ask a few questions about the supply room
in your agency so that you are aware of the requirements related to access and utilization of these items.
    Once you are familiar with the supplies and various forms related
to ongoing documentation, you can devise a system of how the inside
of your car will be organized. Decide how you would like everything to
be situated before asking others how they organize their cars. Doing
things in a new way, or a new paradigm, has a freshness about it. You
view situations differently from the regular staff and this perspective

allows you to explore unique ways of organizing your supplies that you would not have thought about if someone showed you how to do it (Barker, 1997).

Another factor to consider is the climate in which you live. Extremes in temperature are even more severe inside a closed car. Be aware of the effect that variations in temperature can have on your supplies and act accordingly.

Planning Your Day

Call each of your clients to establish the time of the planned visit. Give yourself a range of time. For example, rather than telling the client you will be there at 10 AM, state that you plan to arrive between 9 and 10 AM. This time frame gives you the opportunity to handle unexpected traffic, new developments in a previous client visit, or an emergency.

Quickly ask the client general questions about health status and the equipment and supplies being used in the home. Listen carefully because you may be given information about what you will need during the visit that you may not have anticipated and you can bring those needed supplies with you. For a first visit, this is also an opportunity to clarify directions to the house. Request that any pets, especially those used for protection of the property, be confined during your visit.

Now you are ready to make your home visits. You have all the necessary information about the clients who need to be seen today. Begin your preparations by prioritizing the clients. You may already know the specific times at which certain clients need to be seen. Quickly write this information on a piece of paper. Fill in, by priority and whenever possible by distance, the names of the clients to be seen today.

On your way to a new client, your major concern may be finding the client's residence. The tendency is to focus on your directions, checking for highway or street names and numbers. It is important, at the same time, to be assessing the general environment. Your purpose in doing this is twofold: first, for your personal safety; secondly, it provides data about the impact of the client's environment on his life and his medical condition.

Are the people in the area going about their business in a purposeful way or are there people standing and sitting around? Your safety includes more than the people you see. If you must drive on a road that is full of pot holes, this affects your safety because your car could be damaged. Even with time constraints, you should drive slowly

exercise 8–3

Students in the clinical group are to gather around a map and each student plots out on the map where her client(s) live.

If each of these clients needs to be seen by two or three teams, divide the clients into teams, prioritizing the destinations by distance only.

....

....

....

....

....

and decide carefully how you will navigate the road. Or, as you are driving, you may notice a bee or a bat that has inadvertently gotten into your car. Stop your car and deal with it. Such an incident could cause you harm as well as lead to an accident. Adverse weather and temperature conditions may also call for special precautions.

THE INITIAL VISIT

An initial visit to a client, from start to finish, takes the experienced nurse approximately three hours. This includes establishing rapport, conducting a physical assessment and a home safety assessment, and discussing protocols such as the Patient's Bill of Rights and advance directives. Each activity has accompanying documentation that must be completed during or at the conclusion of the visit.

Because most agencies make the first visit without charge, the first item on your agenda, after introducing yourself, is to determine if the services provided are eligible for reimbursement from Medicare, Medicaid, a health maintenance organization or other insurance company, or if the client is willing to pay out-of-pocket. Medicare "Homebound Status" is determined by the client's ability to ambulate and his level of activity. If no home care coverage is available to the client through the various reimbursement plans, the client is informed of the cost of each visit and given the option of whether or not to continue the visits.

On your arrival at the client's home, a clear introduction of who you are, which agency you represent, and the purpose of the visit are essential. Have your identification card available to show the client, if asked.

In addition to meeting people in the household, you need to assess the immediate environment. Your focus on the client during the introductions greatly facilitates initial rapport. Remember, your degree of caring is communicated mostly on a non-verbal level, so bring yourself back from any distractions in the environment.

Begin by asking the client a general question about his or her health. Listen carefully. Data collection can be facilitated by asking questions that guide the conversation in the direction that gives you the needed health care information. It takes skill to select your words carefully so as to elicit essential data and use your voice to accomplish this objective.

During this process, listen for the client's and family's beliefs and perceptions about the client's disorder or illness, beliefs that include perceived strengths and weaknesses. What is their knowledge base about the illness? How much is the client able to do independently? Who is assuming the primary caregiver role(s)? What are the cultural considerations? What does the medical care consist of and who are the client's physicians and other professionals? Can use of available community resources ease the situation? All of this information unfolds during the visit.

Assessments

The general assessments of community, family, and client are discussed in Chapter. 6. The degree of involvement of the physical assessment depends on the reason for the referral. You need to obtain baseline information related to the amount of assistance needed by the client to perform activities of daily living (ADLs), "homebound" status, and functional status. This information determines the kinds of services needed, the length of service the client requires, and the plan of care.

Many agencies use checklists that include standard assessments that are performed on admission. These assessments include home safety, risk factors for illness, living arrangements, special equipment needs, awareness of client's rights, and establishment of advance directives.

Home Safety

The assessment of the home environment includes awareness of the location of the home in high crime and/or remote areas, structural problems, availability of indoor plumbing and utilities, exposure to heat and cold, lighting, animals, cluttered environment, infestations, food accessibility, and electrical and fire hazards.

Risk Factors

Risk factors such as smoking, alcoholism, obesity, drug dependency and other chronic conditions need to be identified. Social factors such as insufficient household income to manage expenses may become evident and require a referral to a social worker.

 exercise 8-4

This is a group experience.

After each student has written what he or she deems important for assessment in each of the areas of concern listed below, meet as a group and discuss what are safety hazards for each area.

Home Safety Evaluation

Telephone
    Emergency numbers
Ventilation and temperature
Lighting
Electrical
Walking pathways in the home
Condition of stairs and stairwell(s)
Kitchen
Bathroom
Entrances and exits to the dwelling
Stairs
    Outside and inside
Medications
Toxic substances
Fire prevention
Overall evaluation
Other

Living Arrangements

Determination of current living arrangements provides important information about the support system available to the client. Does the client live alone with no assistance or is there outside help? Is there a live-in caregiver, or does the client live with others but not with the caregiver?

 exercise 8–5

A nurse who was working on the weekends for a local home care agency picked up her assignment Friday afternoon. One of the clients, Ms. Allen, had a decubitus on her left little toe. The assignment included specific instructions on wound care and stated that the front door would be unlocked. If the door was locked, the nurse could find the key beneath a flower pot on the front porch.

On Saturday morning, the nurse arrived at Ms. Allen's house, which was in a very quiet, clean housing development. The door was locked. The nurse retrieved the key from under a small green flowerpot and, with trepidation, unlocked the door. The living room was neat but very dusty. The house was dim and quiet. The nurse called out the client's name and there was silence. The nurse twice more called out the client's name as she walked down the shorter corridor to a small room with a light on. In the den was a frail, small lady slumped over in a chair. The television was on but the volume was off. The nurse recalled: "My adrenalin was flowing as I reached out to touch her. Her breathing was easy and unlabored, but her skin was cold as ice till it almost felt moist."

Ms. Allen awakened to the tactile stimulus. A walker was positioned in front of her as if to be used. A plastic bib partially covered with food particles was tied around her neck. The nurse noted that her kyphosis was so severe that she was unable to lift her head very far from her chest. Her hands, as arthritic as they were, lacked the ability to hold and support a cup. A Chux covered her perineum in a diaper fashion and it was drenched with urine. The nurse removed the high top tennis shoes from her feet to perform an assessment and the prescribed wound care. The nurse thought the shoes should not be put back on Ms. Allen's feet, but she replaced them at the client's request.

Ms. Allen answered the nurse's questions in a quivering voice and gave the nurse her reasons for not going into a nursing home. "You just lay there and they don't do anything for you." Ms. Allen had no family support. An aide was coming to the home during the day to feed and bathe her and she received Meals on Wheels twice a day. After the aide left in the afternoon, Ms. Allen remained in that one chair, unable to do anything for herself and was incontinent.

What is your assessment of this client?

....

....

....

....

....

....

What do you think the plan of care for this client focused on?

....

....

....

....

....

....

What would your plan of care include?

....

....

....

....

....

What actions would you take?

....

....

....

....

....

Prioritize:

1. ....

2. ....

3. ....

4. ....

5. ....

Special Equipment or Appliances Used by the Client

Specific types of equipment include dentures, pacemaker, glasses or contact lenses, hearing aid, catheters, oxygen, wheelchair and wheelchair access, cane, walker, hospital bed, bedside commode, and any other special equipment for the shower and/or toilet. Document the names and numbers of equipment vendors and note the condition of these appliances.

The Patient's Bill of Rights

The 1987 Omnibus Budget Reconciliation Act (OBRA) requires home care agencies that participate in the Medicare program to protect and promote the rights of each individual under its care (Haddad & Kapp, 1991). This act led to the development of "Patient/Client Bill of Rights" documents by community based agencies (see the accompanying display). This document also includes patient/client responsibilities for the care provided by the agency and is signed by the client (see the accompanying display).

Advance Directives

The Patient Self-Determination Act is a component of the OBRA Act of 1990. This act requires health care providers to inform patients of their right to make their own health care decisions, including advance directives. An **advance directive** is a legal document created by a men-

CLIENT RIGHTS

Examples of clients' rights to be observed in home care are to:
- Receive dignified and respectful care of person and property
- Trust confidentiality protocols
- Participate in and make decisions about plan of care
- Be notified of type of care, frequency, type of provider, and change in plan of care
- Receive service in a timely manner
- Obtain itemized explanation of charges and reimbursement, including any changes
- Express grievances
- Refuse or discontinue service/equipment
- Be informed of company ownership

From Advanced Home Care, Greensboro, NC.

CLIENT RESPONSIBILITIES

Examples of clients' responsibilities when receiving home care are to:
- Notify agency when not available for service, change of address/phone/insurance status
- Notify agency of any change in conditions or physician
- Notify agency of needed medical equipment repair, when service/equipment is no longer needed, extra equipment needed
- Participate in plan of care
- Meet financial obligations
- Provide accurate, complete health information

From Advanced Home Care, Greensboro, NC.

tally competent adult that provides detailed guidelines about the medical care desired by the client in the event that the client becomes incapable of making those decisions. The **living will** and the **durable power of attorney** are the two most common types of advance directives (Nathanson, 1995).

The living will or "natural death" document allows the person to give specific directions, in advance, about medical treatment in the event of mental incapacity. Remember that living will statutes are not the same in all states (Haddad & Kapp, 1991).

The durable power of attorney for health care is also a legal document. In this document, an individual, known as the principal, appoints an agent or another person to make the medical decisions for him or her in the event of mental incapacity.

"Do not resuscitate" orders are written by the physician and are usually based on discussions that include the client or client substitute and appropriate members of the health care team. These orders withhold or withdraw medical interventions and can be phrased as either "do not resuscitate," "do not hospitalize" and "do not treat" (Haddad & Kapp, 1991).

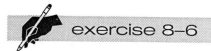

exercise 8–6

Research the Living Will statutes in your state.

In a group discussion, explore your beliefs and feelings when applying these statutes to yourself or to your loved ones.

....

....

....

....

....

....

....

Goal Setting with the Client and Family

Evaluation of the assessments that you conduct creates priorities that can be used to develop a plan of care with the client. The plan of care reflects the medical treatment and nursing and interdisciplinary team interventions. Nursing diagnoses are established and mutual and measurable outcomes are written as short- and long-term goals. These client-centered goals and outcomes provide the direction for the nursing care. A change in priorities for the client's care results in modifications in the goals and outcomes.

Implementation consists of interventions that flow from the plan of care. Interventions and activities are performed by nurses and interdisciplinary team members and begin on the first visit. They include performing nursing measures, teaching knowledge and skills to the client and/or caregiver, and providing referrals to appropriate community resources. Changes in the plan of care result from client, caregiver, and/or health care team members' input. This collaboration results in an effective plan of care.

INFECTION CONTROL

The same principles that apply to infection control in the hospital apply to community based agencies and home settings. Some of the facts may vary, but the end result is the same. For example, there are many different kinds of organisms that exist in the hospital and patients are continuously at risk for nosocomial infections. Any one that goes into that environment is at risk. In the home, this situation is usually reversed. Most homes do not contain numerous pathogenic organisms. Organisms are most often brought into the home either by the client through infectious agents related to the illness or by the nurse and other visitors.

Your technique greatly decreases the types and numbers of organisms transferred from one environment to another. **Standard Precautions,** which include Universal Precautions and were instituted in 1995, are the same for community based nursing as they are for hospital nursing. The only differences may be in their application. A reminder of the basic principle behind standard precautions is that every client must be treated as if he or she has a communicable disease.

Many procedures performed in the hospital using sterile technique are frequently down graded to **clean technique** in the home setting. In changing dressings on wounds in the home, the decision may be made to use clean gloves and dressings instead of sterile ones; this would not happen in treating the same wound in the hospital. Another example of a change in technique may be found with the client who has learned to catheterize herself. The technique is clean rather than sterile.

The following measures are used to limit the spread of organisms from one person or place to another.

Bag Technique

The nurse carries many of the basic supplies inside a nursing bag. The inside of the nursing bag is considered clean. Every effort is made to prevent cross-contamination from home to home and client to client. Until recently, public health nurses carried newspaper with them on home visits and when there was not a clean place to put the nursing bag, it was placed on a piece of newspaper. Since this practice is no longer followed, a Chux or piece of disposable plastic is used as a place to put the bag in an unclean situation. Place the bag on something rather than using the floor.

Remember, you are in the client's home and you must ask permission to look for specific items or to go from one room to another for whatever you need. Once you have the client's permission to wash your hands in the appropriate place, open your bag. You packed the liquid soap and papertowels at the top of the bag, so take what you need, then close the bag. Wash your hands thoroughly. Now your hands are clean and you can freely move within the bag to retrieve whatever you need. Then reclose the bag. If you need to reenter the bag, wash your hands again to keep the inside clean.

You will continuously be using your judgment while delivering care in the home. If you enter a very unclean environment or there is no running water, use your hand cleaner (gel, lotion, or wipes). Since bar soap and cloth towels harbor organisms even in a clean setting, use your own washing and drying materials.

Handwashing

Handwashing is essential before client contact, during contact if needed, and at the completion of the visit. After you remove your gloves, wash your hands. Remember to change your gloves between procedures and whenever you think it is necessary. If you must use a cleaner without running water because of the circumstances, wash your hands as soon as possible at the next opportunity.

Supplies required by OSHA

You'll have Occupational Safety and Health Administration (OSHA) required supplies with you to use as needed. These supplies include:

- Gloves
- Masks, aprons, eye shields
- Sharps container
- Plastic bag (for double-bagging)
- Airway shields
- Handcleaners, papertowels
- Clean-up supplies for spills
- Disinfectants

Care of Your Equipment

Before you leave your car, decide on the equipment and supplies that will be needed during the visit. These items are all you bring into the home. Once equipment enters the home, it must be cleaned according to agency protocols before it is removed from that environment. For example, before leaving the home, wipe the entire diaphragm/bell of your stethoscope and wipe the cover on your sphygmomanometer. Unused supplies are not to be brought out of the house and restocked in your car; leave them in the home or discard them, if appropriate. For instructions about cleaning and disinfecting specific equipment, review both the manufacturers' guidelines for the equipment and your agency's policies and procedure manual.

Containing the Spread of Infection

If you have a cold or an infection and you enter the client's home, you are unnecessarily exposing the client and the family to those organisms. The same is true of visitors who come to the house. If the client's immune system is compromised, then the caregiver and family need to remind visitors of the consequences of exposure to infections. Caregivers who are stressed and overworked may be especially vulnerable to organisms being introduced into the environment.

If the client is a source of pathogenic organisms, it is important to teach the family/caregiver what to do to prevent the transmission of organisms. Knowledge about the diagnosis includes how organisms are transmitted. You need to remind the caregiver that, whenever he or she comes in contact with the client's body fluids or blood, gloves need to be worn. Teach the caregiver how to properly remove the gloves and reinforce correct handwashing technique.

Proper handwashing also needs to be taught to the client/caregiver. Conduct a demonstration and have the persons involved give a return demonstration. If they know the reasons why proper handwashing is needed, they are more likely to comply with this action. The same is true for teaching the use and disposal of gloves. Clients/caregivers may want to reuse gloves in an attempt to be economical and/or because "they're not dirty".

DOCUMENTATION AND RECORDKEEPING

This section examines when and where you do your documentation rather than the content (which is addressed in Chapter 4). Most agencies require that the paperwork on client visits be submitted within 24 hours. The time and place in which you decide to prepare your documentation is variable and depends on your preferences and schedule. Examples of different approaches are discussed below.

First, no matter when you prepare your records, it helps to jot down notes about pertinent information while you are with the client. This is especially true in the case of data such as blood pressure and wound measurements.

To decide on the best time to do your paperwork, it may help to look at the broader picture. You work hard during the day to assist clients with their problems and must frequently practice under significant time constraints. As a result, you may not think you have time to document your care until after work hours, usually at home. If incomplete paperwork hangs over your head all evening and you are not able to work on it until family members are in bed, you may want to take a hard look at this. A real disadvantage to completing the records later is that you may have to take a few moments to sort out the details related to a particular family from all the others. Details that earlier in the day were clear can be lost with time.

As an alternative to preparing your records at night, consider documenting each visit shortly after it is concluded. After you leave the client, you get into your car, drive a short distance, pull over (if it is safe, of course) and do your recordkeeping. The information you need for your charting is still clear in your mind and writing it up takes only a few minutes. With all your records up to date, including your mileage record, you drive to your next visit. As you proceed through the day, most if not all of your documentation is complete. If something out of the ordinary is incomplete, it will not take you long to complete it at the office. Finishing your paperwork at the office at the end of the day, if that is convenient, gives you a chance to submit the appropriate records and do miscellaneous tasks such as filing. In addition, you can make a note of the supplies you need to restock in your car for the next day. When you leave for the day, you are free until the next day. Many nurses are then able to restore themselves in the evening. You will need to choose the method of documentation that is most practical and comfortable for you.

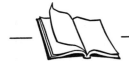

CHAPTER HIGHLIGHTS

1. The delivery of home care poses additional concerns about confidentiality due to the accessibility to sensitive information about clients.

2. Preparation for the initial visit encompasses considering your personal safety, organizing your equipment and supplies, and planning your day.

3. The initial visit includes conducting assessments and setting goals and expected outcomes.

4. Infection control measures are based on the same principles as those used in the hospital. Those that apply to home care include bag technique, handwashing, transporting supplies required by OSHA, and care of your equipment.

5. The nurse has some flexibility in choosing when and where she does her documentation.

REFERENCES

Barker, J. (1997). *Paradigm Mastery Series.* (Videos). St. Paul, MN: Star Thrower Distribution Corp.

Haddad, A.M. and Kapp, M.B. (1991). *Ethical and Legal Issues in Home Health Care.* Norwalk, CT: Appleton & Lange.

Nathanson, M.D. (1995). *Home Health Care Answer Book: Legal Issues for Providers.* Rockville, MD: Aspen.

9.

Community Based Care Settings

Professional nurses have practiced in community settings since 1877 when the first graduate nurses began to visit patients in their homes. Prior to that time, lay people provided home care. Since then, professional nurses have been employed in various community based settings on a consistent basis as these settings emerged. Traditional settings included local health departments, home care, schools, and industry. After World War II, patients came to physicians' offices rather than the physician attending to the patient at home, thus creating the need for more office nurses. As health clinics opened, nurses were hired to provide patient care. Hospice agencies were established in the United States in the 1970s. Today, a variety of health care centers are commonplace and include rehabilitation, rural health, retirement, and nursing centers. Contemporary problems have led to other creative solutions in care delivery such as assisted living facilities, parish nursing, and nurses in independent practice.

This chapter briefly discusses many of these community based settings and the type of nursing care provided by each, beginning with the traditional settings and ending with contemporary settings.

TRADITIONAL CARE SETTINGS

Traditional settings are those settings that came into existence around 1900. They include local health departments, home care agencies, school health nursing, and occupational health nursing.

Local Health Departments

Local health departments, which are tax-supported, employ public health nurses to deliver nursing care to various population groups. Although a baccalaureate degree in nursing is preferred as an entry requirement for this setting because of the foundation of public health theory and practice that is taught in these programs, the majority of public health nurses are prepared in diploma and associate degree programs.

Organization and roles of public health nurses vary within local health departments. In some counties, nurses are assigned to a geographic area and function as generalists who provide nursing care to clients and families who live within that jurisdiction. Nurses in other local health departments are specialists in areas such as geriatrics, pediatrics, or maternity and provide care to clients in need of these services. The major emphasis of public health nurses is prevention and education.

The services of the health department focus on the public's health and are available to everyone although there may be a sliding fee scale of payment. These services are delivered through the establishment of specialized clinics whose formation is determined on the basis of the problems present in a community. Clinics that offer screening and treatment for diseases that threaten the health of the community, such as tuberculosis or sexually transmitted diseases, are mandated by each state. Depending on the services that a community decides are important, local health departments can maintain clinics for family planning, maternal/child health, adult health, immuniza-

 exercise 9–1

You are the public health nurse who has a referral to visit a 6-month-old infant of a mother with Down syndrome in order to assess the infant for developmental delays.

A home visit is made. You interview the maternal grandmother who is caring for the infant. Subjective data:

"I don't know where she (the mother) is"; "I don't know what is in the bottle"; "I'm not sure how many wet or dirty diapers he has had."

Objective data: large 6-month-old infant alone on couch; no crib or playpen; yellow fluid in baby bottle (unidentified); mother not present, only maternal grandmother and maternal great grandmother in the home; no developmental toys or interaction; no telephone; no reading materials or writing implements in view.

In addition to the above subjective and objective data, what other assessments would you need and want to conduct?

....

....

....

....

....

....

Based on these assessments, what are your priorities in this situation?

....

....

....

....

....

....

What is your plan of care for this client?

....

....

....

....

....

....

....

tions, and screenings. In addition to their practice within clinics, many public health nurses may work at other sites such as prisons, wellness centers, workplaces, congregate feeding sites, Head Start programs, and shelters for the homeless.

In many areas throughout the United States, health departments provide home care services. Enhanced practice has been extended to many public health nurses through additional education. In areas where there are shortages of primary caregivers, these nurses conduct health screenings required by Medicaid and dispense drugs from a public health formulary. The major focus of public health nursing is prevention and education.

Home Care Agencies

The fastest growing segment of health care is home care. Currently, there are more than 1800 home care agencies operating in the United States. They are an extension of hospital care and are based on the medical paradigm. The care is on a periodic rather than a 24 hour per day basis that is delivered to the client at home, usually during scheduled visits (see Chapter 8 for a discussion about preparing for home visits). This care is comprehensive and holistic, includes the family, and uses a multidisciplinary approach for the purposes of promoting, maintaining, and restoring health. Depending on the agency, the home care nurse may either visit clients within a designated geographic area and provide general medical/surgical nursing care or may deliver specialized nursing care to a designated population such as pediatric clients. In 1993, a certification examination for the generalist level of practice in home care became available, through which nurses can establish their competency in this setting.

School Nursing

The problems related to communicable diseases and truancy led to the development of school health nursing in the early 1900s. The role of the school health nurse has emerged over time, and was designed according to the needs of school-age children. The political climate and federal and state legislation have a great influence on the role of school health. State laws and mandates determine the type of services needed in a school and these vary from state to state.

School health nurses are employed by the local health department in some states and by individual school districts in others. Many schools provide comprehensive health care services that are provided by volunteer physicians, a school nurse, social worker, nutritionist, and lay volunteers. The multidisciplinary team can also include the principal and teachers

The roles of the school health nurse include health education, health services, and environmental health. The practice of the school health nurse is based on all three levels of prevention with an emphasis on primary prevention and the promotion of health and safety of both the students and the school environment. The nurse conducts screenings, provides emergency and first-aid care, maintains records, offers individual and group health counseling, makes referrals, directs needs assessments and research, and works with the community on school issues.

In order to be proficient in this setting, the school health nurse must have a strong knowledge base in public and school law, school health administration and program management, health education, counseling, first aid, and growth and development. The American Nurses Association and the National Association of School Nurses offer certification examinations in school health nursing.

Occupational Health Nursing

Occupational health nursing is a nursing specialty that focuses on the health and safety of workers in the workplace and on the workplace as a setting. It is population oriented, meaning that the services and programs are directed to the entire workforce as well as to needs of indi-

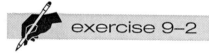

exercise 9–2

The school health nurse meets weekly with a group of high risk female students at a local middle school, grades 6–8 (ages 12–14). High risk factors include: adolescent pregnancy, illegitimacy, abortion, truancy, smoking, unprotected sexual activity, suspension from school, drug abuse, unstable home environment, and/or low socioeconomic status.

Ground rules for the weekly meetings are: one person talks at a time; open communication; nurse can give advice; and confidentiality is stressed. The students openly discuss having unprotected sex with multiple partners and taking drugs. They also state that they hope to go to college.

If you were the school nurse, to be effective, what would you have to believe about these girls?

....
....
....
....
....
....

What do you think the girls believe about themselves?

....
....
....
....
....
....

What would your goals be for this group?

....
....
....
....
....
....

How would you communicate your goals?

....
....
....
....
....
....
....

What would your plan include?

....

....

....

....

....

vidual employees and their dependents. The occupational health nurse (OHN) is a company's prime resource for issues related to health care and for the delivery of health services.

The first occupational health nurse, Betty Moulder, was hired by a group of coal mining companies in Pennsylvania in 1888. From that time until today, the practice of occupational health nursing has changed dramatically as a result of both changes in our social, economic, and political structures and specific factors such as technological advances, health care reform, and managed care.

This setting is guided by a number of laws and regulations that are administered by various federal agencies that the OHN, in the role of manager, must be knowledgeable about and apply in her practice. They include:

- *Occupational Safety and Health Act* (OSH Act, Public Law 91-596, 1970). A federal agency within the Department of Labor, Occupational Safety and Health Administration (OSHA), was established to provide for the safety and health of the workplace by enacting, administering and enforcing the approved standards.

- *Drug-Free Workplace Act* of 1988.

- *Department of Transportation Drug and Alcohol Testing*. This act requires alcohol and drug testing of employees in the aviation, railroad, mass transit, and motor carrier industries. Prevention programs were mandated in 1994.

- *Americans with Disabilities Act* of 1990 (ADA). Persons with disabilities who are qualified and seek employment with companies cannot be discriminated against on the basis of their disabilities.

- *Family and Medical Leave Act* (FMLA), 1993. This act requires employers to provide up to 12 weeks of unpaid leave in any 12 month period for: the birth of a child; adoption or foster care; serious illness of a parent, spouse or child; or serious illness of the employee.

- *Equal Employment Opportunity Commission* (EEOC), Title VII of the 1964 Civil Rights Act, went into effect in 1965 and is responsible for legislation related to drug use, disabilities, and affirmative action in the workplace.

- *The Environmental Protection Agency* (EPA), which protects water and air quality, was established in 1970.
- *Workers' Compensation.* Each state has established workers' compensation statutes that provide monetary compensation to employees who are injured on their jobs.

The health of a company's workforce and whether or not the employees are medically able to perform their assigned work is a major responsibility of the OHN. This is accomplished through the roles of:

1. *Educator:* conducts programs on hazards in the workplace, wellness programs, and employee assistance programs on mental health and personal problems.
2. *Clinician:* provides nursing care for work and non-work related injuries and illnesses, performs case management, and conducts biologic monitoring for identification of exposure, such as blood samples for lead levels.
3. *Consultant:* functions as a member of an interdisciplinary team and works with management on various issues such as ergonomics for cumulative trauma disorders and recognition and control of hazards.

The expansion of United States markets into the global economy extends the responsibilities of the OHN to include immunizations, pre-travel health history and physical examinations, health and safety education for travel, and post-travel physical examinations.

The professional organization for occupational health nurses is the American Association of Occupational Health Nurses, Inc. (AAOHN). This organization defines the scope and standards for occupational

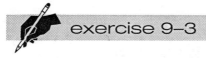

exercise 9–3

An employee who worked as a spinner on the first shift for 25 years, came to the nurse with a chief complaint of weight loss, fatigue, weakness, and congestion. The nurse referred her to the plant physician who referred her to her family physician. She was hospitalized because her hemoglobin was very low. She was tested for tuberculosis and the results were positive for pulmonary tuberculosis.

What are the responsibilities of the plant to the employees? What steps are to be taken?

....

....

....

....

....

....

Who, if anyone, would need to be tested for tuberculosis?

....

....

....

....

....

....

What is your rationale?

....

....

....

....

....

....

How do you handle questions by the media, if they arise?

....

....

....

....

....

....

health nursing and provides professional credentialing and certification in occupational health nursing.

PHYSICIAN-DIRECTED SETTINGS

Community based settings that developed around the 1950s were established largely by physicians and were based on the medical model. These settings include physicians' offices and out-patient and other clinics.

Physicians' Offices

As physicians began treating patients in their offices on a regular basis instead of making home visits, a subsequent need for nurses to care for those patients was created. Nurses play a vital role within these settings by assisting, assessing, and teaching the patient during the office visit. In addition, nurses make important assessments while talking with patients who call the office with health concerns. Today, specialty nurses who are employed by physicians in office environments may triage patients, teach classes to groups of patients, and visit patients who are admitted to the hospital. Care that requires high-tech interventions is also included in the office nurse's practice. As the number of physicians within a practice increases, so does the number of generalist and specialty nurses. The responsibility these nurses incur within this setting also increases.

Out-Patient and Other Clinics

During the 1950s, as physicians decreased the number of patients they treated at home, out-patient clinics also emerged. These settings were designed for patients who did not need to be hospitalized in order to receive specialized services which were delivered on an out-patient basis. These services included patient teaching, dressing changes, irrigations, injections, and diagnostic testing. Specialty clinics that focus on areas such as prenatal assessment developed in response to similar needs.

Today, services provided in out-patient facilities include day surgery and many advanced procedures. The role of the nurse in these settings is often identical to that performed in the hospital; for example, a recovery room nurse. The nursing care in these facilities can include pre- and post-operative care and related patient education.

CONTEMPORARY SETTINGS

Contemporary settings are those settings that have evolved in the last 20 or 30 years. The services provided in these settings may have been available previously, but were either unstructured, informal, or incorporated into other services. For example, before the 1960s, a family caring for a member who was dying or who required rehabilitation services did not have access to the formal settings in the community that are available today.

There are many types of community based agencies and services that provide care for clients discharged from acute care facilities and others that admit clients on an out-patient basis. The number and kinds of agencies depend on the needs, priorities, and resources of a particular community. These settings include hospice care, rehabilitation centers, homeless and indigent care clinics, elder care facilities, mental health clinics, parish nursing, rural health centers, and nursing centers.

Hospice Care

Hospice provides care to the dying. To be eligible for this care, a client must be judged to be within six months of death. The care can be given in homes, hospitals, extended care facilities, or adult day care centers. The goal of hospice is to provide care, support, and education to the terminally ill and their families.

Today, more than 2,100 hospices nationwide provide hospice care that includes 24-hour coverage, access to an interdisciplinary health care team, the use of volunteers, symptom management, bereavement services, education of caregivers, and respite care. Currently, a case is being made for an expansion of the six-month eligibility rule to include clients with high impact diagnoses regardless of their choice of treatment (Ryndes, 1995).

Hospice agencies must be licensed by the state in which they are located and certified by the Health Care Financing Administration in order to be covered by Medicare and other third party payers. Hospice is cost-effective and was the first managed care benefit of Medicare. There are many sites on the World Wide Web where information about hospice is available.

Rehabilitation Centers

Rehabilitation services are provided in many community based settings and focus on the process of restoring an individual to a maximal level of independence after experiencing a disabling illness or injury. Rehabilitation centers provide acute care for clients with emotional and/or physical disabilities.

The rehabilitation nurse is a clinician who gives direct care, has excellent assessment and counseling skills, and conducts teaching that includes primary, secondary, and tertiary prevention. An example of a specialty area within rehabilitation nursing is care of clients with spinal cord injuries. The certified rehabilitation registered nurse (CRRN) examination is given by the Rehabilitation Nursing Certificate Board (RNCB).

Subacute care is usually provided on a short-term basis. An example is a client who has had a hip replacement. Before the establishment of Diagnosis Related Groups, a patient who underwent a hip replacement would remain in the hospital to complete a series of physical or occupational therapy treatments. This patient is now being discharged earlier to the community. In the event that an adequate support system is absent in the home and services are reimbursable through Medicare, this client can be discharged to an extended care facility that provides the necessary care and physical therapy measures. The prescribed treatments are carried out in this setting until the client is ready to be discharged to the home. Home care nursing visits may then be necessary for follow-up until the client has completely recovered.

Homeless and Indigent Care Clinics

Many large communities have clinics, such as the Urban Ministries, that serve the homeless and indigent populations. Small amounts of federal funds are available through Title 11 of the Stewart B. McKinney Assistance Act of 1987 (P.L.100-77) to supplement the work of these agencies. These clinics are often operated by health care professionals, such as physicians, nurses, dentists, and social workers who volunteer on a regular basis. Very few of the staff members are salaried. Fees for services are on a sliding scale. In addition, Medicare and Medicaid are billed when appropriate.

Elder Care Facilities

As the population ages, more retirement centers and communities are being built. **Retirement centers** provide several levels of services: independent living, assisted living, and skilled nursing facilities. In centers that provide all three levels, people of retirement age who are independent enter as residents and are offered apartment-style living arrangements. As these residents require medical and nursing care, they move to the second and possibly the third levels. In larger centers, nurses may work in all three levels; for example, the practice of a nurse working with the independent residents would include assessing health concerns, teaching, directing programs, and performing screenings.

Retirement communities usually consist of secure condominium and apartment living. To assist with basic health care needs, physicians may have offices on the property and a nurse may be available to the residents. Other levels of care are usually not available.

Adult day care centers enable elderly people to stay with their families and avoid being admitted to nursing homes or extended care facilities. In addition, the services administered by these centers provide respite for the caregivers and permit many of them to continue to work. Adult day care centers provide older adults with regular meals, prescribed medications, safety, rest, social interaction, and stimulation from programs that involve children and pets. These centers are very cost-effective and extremely beneficial to older adults and their families.

Long-term care facilities or nursing homes provide services for clients who do not need hospitalization but, rather, skilled nursing care. These facilities provide medical care, full-time nursing care, and various types of therapy such as occupational and physical. Residents are physically and/or mentally incapacitated and can be of any age, although most residents are elderly.

Assisted living facilities provide assistance with activities of daily living such as taking medications, bathing, dressing, and eating. These facilities are developed to be as much like home as possible and residents have their own bedrooms. A person must be sufficiently independent to meet the criteria for admission to these facilities. A nurse is not usually on site; however, nursing may be available on a consultant basis.

Mental Health Clinics

As patients with mental conditions and diseases, who would have been hospitalized in the past, were discharged from mental institutions into the community, the need for boarding homes and mental health clinics increased. Boarding homes provide living in a home environment for people unable to live independently. Nursing care is not provided in these facilities. Nursing practice in mental health clinics consists of

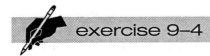

exercise 9–4

When a person is admitted to a psychiatric unit, it is standard protocol for the nurse to thoroughly check and identify any property that the client possesses for labelling and storage.

A very disheveled, physically strong, middle-aged man was admitted to the clinic from the street. He gently placed his tattered brown suitcase, held together by a belt, onto the table. As the nurse unfastened the belt and opened the latches, she expected to find several bunched up articles of clothing. To her surprise, the suitcase was filled with a ten pound bag of raw potatoes.

Four days later, as the client was discharged to the street, his concern was not about his medications or follow-up care at the mental clinic, but that his potatoes be returned to him.

As a student in the mental health clinic:

What are your beliefs about this client?

....

....

....

....

....

....

How would this information guide your approach to this client?

....

....

....

....

....

....

What would your assessment include?

....

....

....

....

....

How would you proceed with your care?

....

....

....

....

....

monitoring medications, leading group therapy, performing diagnostic testing, and conducting client assessments that include the need for hospitalization.

Parish Nursing

A parish nurse practices within a church congregation. This concept began in the 1960s as churches began to hire nurses to provide preventive and holistic care to members of their congregations. There are a variety of structures and practice opportunities for parish nursing. For instance, nurses may provide care on a volunteer basis, several small churches may join together to hire a nurse, or several nurses can share a church. The most formalized structure within parish nursing is the institutional model. In this model, an institution, such as a hospital, retirement center, nursing home, university, or community health agency may sponsor a Parish Nurse Program. The nurse is then employed by the institution.

A parish nurse needs to possess those characteristics required for community based nursing in any setting, including autonomy, flexibility, effective communication skills, self-confidence, and a strong knowledge base. The one characteristic unique to parish nursing is spiritual maturity, which is reflected in a strong sense of who the nurse is and her relationship to God. It is not necessary that the nurse be a member of a particular denomination in order to practice parish nursing; however, the spiritual component is required.

Parish nurses work with members of the congregation in the roles of clinician, educator, counselor, referral source and liaison with community resources, facilitator and teacher of volunteers and interpreter of the close relationship between faith and health (Djupe et al, 1991).

The church provides support to the parish nurse usually in the form of a work space with furnishings, equipment, secretarial support, and educational materials. The parish nurse agrees to carry malpractice insurance, keep statistical records, communicate with the pastor and church staff on a regular basis, and attend various support and educational sessions (Djupe et al, 1991).

Large institutions such as hospitals that sponsor parish nursing programs expect that client referrals by the nurse will be made to the hospital for services such as diagnostic work-ups, out-patient clinics, and emergency room visits. The referral process is facilitated by the networking done by the parish nurse. Questions about the institutional model of parish nursing can be answered by calling the National Parish Nurse Resource Center of the Lutheran General Health Care System at 708-MY NURSE (708-696-8773).

Rural Health Centers

Rural living poses unique health care problems that the nurse needs to consider. People in rural areas may live great distances from health care facilities and transportation to these facilities may be unavailable. This isolation supports a lifestyle of independence and attempts to take care of problems alone or on the basis of a neighbor's advice. Within a small population, people are known well to each other and the issues of privacy and trust become significant. Newcomers to the community can have difficulty overcoming these barriers.

In rural populations, medical care is often sought only in a crisis. The injuries suffered in farming communities, however, are serious and lack of accessible medical care often leads to fatalities. The autonomous lifestyle can make primary prevention and health promotion difficult for residents to accept.

These issues and the lack of adequate medical care in rural areas led to the passage of the Rural Health Clinic Services Act in 1977 that created both the Community Health Center Program and Migrant Health Centers whose purposes are to provide health care services to these populations. Federal funds are allocated for the delivery of health care to rural areas and include indirect reimbursement for nurse practitioners (NPs) and physicians' assistants (PAs), which means that rural health centers are reimbursed directly and the money is used to pay the salaries of these professionals. Managed care companies currently view rural areas as being the next expanding market for their services.

The rural health centers are operated with a multidisciplinary team approach and the staff includes physicians, PAs, nurses, NPs, laboratory technicians, and outreach workers. Preventive dental care is also provided. Other features of these centers may be extended hours in the evenings and on weekends and use of a trauma room so treatment can begin before emergency medical personnel arrive. These centers have formal and informal linkages for services with other community agencies such as surrounding hospitals, local health departments, county home care agencies, shelters for battered women, and other rural health care centers.

Nursing Centers

Nursing centers are managed by nurses. Advanced practice nurses (APNs) often collaborate with other nurses and community members in these independent facilities (Stanhope & Lancaster, 1996). Student nurses may also have clinical experiences in nursing centers. Because of the variations among nurse practice acts and other laws in different states, an APN in one state can independently prescribe certain medications in that state but not in another. In addition to the specific laws that govern nursing practice, the needs of a particular population or community can determine the type of center that is developed.

Managed care presents a challenge to nursing centers by creating highly competitive environments. Nursing information systems are currently collecting data that will be used to compare nursing-based care to other practices including managed care in the areas of cost and outcomes. This analysis should demonstrate the effectiveness of the care delivered by nursing centers to specific populations.

In addition to the establishment of nursing centers, other creative solutions to health care delivery issues are being sought by nurses. For example, nurses are exploring ways to ensure that clients receive the care they need in spite of their inability to pay for these services. In Pennsylvania, three schools of nursing collaborated with a home care agency to assign nursing students to caseloads that consisted of clients whose nursing care was no longer reimbursable. As a result, clients received excellent care and were able to be readmitted to reimbursable care if their conditions changed (Tucker et al, 1996).

exercise 9-5

What are your beliefs about a situation in which a client continues to need care, the source of payment is discontinued, the client is unable to pay for services and the agency discharges the client?

1. ....
   ....
   ....
   ....
   ....

2. ....
   ....
   ....
   ....

3. ....
   ....
   ....
   ....
   ....

With a partner, exchange your beliefs on this subject.

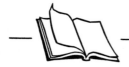

CHAPTER HIGHLIGHTS

1. Community based settings are numerous, varied and growing in numbers. They provide an entire range of practice settings for nurses.

2. Local health departments, home care agencies, school nursing, and occupational settings have been in existence for about 100 years and have changed dramatically over time.

3. Physicians' offices and numerous expanded clinics provide diversified settings for community based nurses.

4. Contemporary settings continue to develop and provide opportunities for practice for community based nurses. These settings include hospice care, rehabilitation centers, homeless and indigent care clinics, elder care facilities, mental health clinics, parish nursing, rural health centers, and nursing centers.

REFERENCES

Djupe, A.M., Olson, H., Ryan, J., and Lantz, J.C. (1991). *An Institutionally Based Model of Parish Nursing Services.* Park Ridge, IL: National Parish Nurse Resource Center.

Ryndes, T. (1995). New beginnings in hospice. *Healthcare Forum Journal* 38(2): 27–29.

Stanhope, M. and Lancaster, J. (1996). *Community Health Nursing.* (4th ed.) St. Louis, MO: Mosby.

Tucker, M., Nester, P., Gross, E., and Johnstone, S. (1996). Increasing student home health care experiences: the client wins. *Home Healthcare Nurse* 14(1): 33–38.

10.

Future Trends

The chaos and confusion we feel and see today in the health care system are the result of changes at the core of the system rather than the usual superficial modifications. A shift of values and beliefs is being created from both within and outside this environment. The effect of these changes is causing an expansion of activity in community based nursing and a contraction of the need for nurses in acute care settings. This movement, coupled with awesome technological changes, is creating an environment that is exciting and, at the same time, frightening. One can only speculate at this point about the final transformation of the health care system. However, we can examine the direction of present changes and wonder what nursing practice will be like in just a few short years. A few of these speculations are discussed below.

INFORMATION TECHNOLOGY

The technology for sharing information about clients will eventually be available to all health care practitioners. For example, in the rural community of Shelby, North Carolina, the local health department, the home care agency, and the local hospitals formed a corporation to serve the community. This led to collaboration among the local physicians, nurses, nurse practitioners, health department, and other health care personnel. A computerized system that maintains the health record of each client being cared for in the county was purchased by the corporation.

This arrangement is clearly having a positive impact by providing cost-effective, quality health care to the county's residents. When a patient is seen by another agency within the corporation (for example, at the hospital emergency room on a weekend), the appropriate hospital personnel are able to access the patient's central record on the computer, even if this patient has never been seen at the hospital. Health care providers are able to instantly obtain health information about the client without each provider asking the same questions over and over. Immediate access to pertinent information can increase decision making skills, make the patient feel better cared for, and improve collaboration of team members.

Optical disks, which are able to store a significantly larger amount of data than is possible on hard drives, will be used as floppy disks are used today. Voice communication will make it possible for the nurse in community based practice to talk into her computer to record and retrieve information (Swansburg, 1997). It is easy to envision the home care nurse, through voice communication, recording her assessments and receiving several options for teaching strategies from the computer. The chosen option would then be immediately printed out. Nursing care plans and critical pathways will be available and accessible at any given moment.

Legal and ethical questions about the availability of client information are primarily centered on confidentiality. Who has access to which information needs to be addressed continuously. Strategies for handling these issues need to be in place and frequently monitored.

Information technology will also help to make health information readily available to consumers. This trend would create a closer partnership between the health care provider and the client. If the client is able to participate in his care, this would lead to more self-responsibility. Information technology will be used to compile biostatistics related to client contacts with health care providers. It is envisioned that providers and consumers will have access to the synthesis of this information, which will result in health information about the community as a whole. Knowledge of which communities are at risk for specific diseases and conditions will be at the practitioner's fingertips.

The Internet is opening all kinds of avenues for the sharing of information on both intradisciplinary and interdisciplinary levels. The continuous expansion and explosion of new technologies is creating greater accessibility to facts and information and data from journals, indices, and university courses. Conversations among professionals that include visuals will become commonplace.

THE IMPACT OF COST CONTAINMENT ON NURSING EDUCATION

Managed care is here to stay. The paradigm of nursing that focuses on caring with no involvement in the cost of care is antiquated. The new paradigm that establishes a balance between caring and costing has replaced the traditional paradigm. Nursing is still in the process of learning to view the phenomenon of caring and costing as a positive configuration. Changes in nursing curriculums based on this new paradigm are in response to a major demand for cost containment from payors.

PREVENTION

Principles and concepts established by the public health sciences will eventually be incorporated into managed care. Today, managed care systems within the community based setting are active mainly on the secondary and tertiary levels of care. Within this structure of prevention, specified amounts of care at a designated cost are provided to clients with diagnosed medical problems. In an effort to keep people healthy in a cost-effective way, great value in the form of reimbursement will eventually be placed on health and wellness promotion and primary prevention. Attention will be placed on identifying and minimizing risk factors that are considered deleterious to health. Positive lifestyle changes will be rewarded. There will be a seamless blend of public health and community based care. More and more nurses, employed by health maintenance organizations and other managed care organizations, will be making home visits to clients to support primary and secondary prevention strategies in an effort to decrease health care costs.

With the focus on primary prevention, entire industries that support negative habits, such as the tobacco industry, could disappear. As the government and other payors decide what is best for the majority through availability of payment, individual rights can become endangered. The consequences of these decisions are complicated and are difficult to separate. For example, the targeting of children in cigarette advertisements and the manipulation of the amount of nicotine to get more smokers addicted is grossly unethical on the part of the tobacco companies. However, it is one thing to go after the companies for such behavior and it is quite another to work towards the elimination of the industry because it is "bad."

Do adults have the right to choose whether or not to smoke? This question is further complicated when one asks: "Who will pay the bill for the deleterious effects of smoking on a person's health?" When actions are taken in response to the cost of care that eliminate individual rights, we as a nation are in serious trouble. Where do we draw the line? Will liquor companies and breweries be targeted for health reasons? Will companies that produce non-nutritious foods be the subject of scrutiny and criticism? These issues are very complex and enmeshed in our collective beliefs. As public policy continues to support group rights as opposed to individual rights, it creates a shift in outcomes that has far-reaching consequences for everyone. Decisions made by the federal and state legislatures and the Supreme Court create changes that dramatically affect how we live our lives.

COLLABORATION IN HEALTH CARE

In the past, the cohesiveness within each group of health care providers supported competition rather than collaboration. In order to survive today, health care providers and various agencies are learning to collaborate and work together in creative ways. This cooperation fosters change and strengthens the fabric of the system, improves client care, and restores a sense of stability. The strength that is created by collaboration actually keeps the organization functioning on a high level that, in turn, keeps competition at a distance.

NURSING PRACTICE IN COMMUNITY BASED NURSING

Let us compare nursing practice in both home care and hospice settings. Currently, home care nurses basically practice the same type of nursing that is performed in the hospital. The purpose of a home care nursing visit is to monitor a client who has a specific medical need. The focus is on the client and most often involves care of physical needs such as dressing and catheter changes, monitoring and administration of medications, and teaching that is related to the condition or disease. Care is intermittent or part-time. The services of volunteers are not used. The physician is responsible for the plan of care.

In contrast, hospice functions quite differently from home care for many reasons. The most important factor is that the client is judged to be within six months of death and the administration of aggressive treatment has ceased. The physician relinquishes care of the client to hospice, except for medical orders related to pain medications and other palliative measures. Nursing assumes the role of coordinating the care. There is a focus not only on the client but on the family as well. The care is comprehensive, administered by a multidisciplinary team, and includes responses to physical, emotional, and spiritual needs. Volunteers receive specialized training and provide a valuable service. In addition, there is 24-hour nursing coverage. A major emphasis is on "celebrating" the client's life. After the client's death, one year of bereavement counseling is available to the family.

If you were to compare home care nursing with hospice, you would discover that hospice care is quite similar to the services traditionally provided by public health nurses. It is holistic in nature. In light of the differences between the two practice settings, several questions are raised. Doesn't everyone, especially sick people, have spiritual needs? Why is this aspect deemed important only when one is about to die? Wouldn't it be an excellent idea for everyone to celebrate their life every day rather than celebrating it only when a person is close to death? Couldn't anyone who is sick benefit from the services of a volunteer, especially in situations in which the caregiver is provided with a reprieve from their duties?

 exercise 10–1

What would a society or culture have to believe in order to decide that hospice services should only be available to the dying and not to the chronically sick or to those who will recover?

....

....

....

....

....

....

....

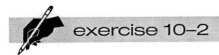

exercise 10–2

What would our society have to believe in order to model home care agencies after hospice?

....

....

....

....

....

What changes would have to be made?

....

....

....

....

....

ADVANCED PRACTICE NURSING

In an effort to contain health care costs, innovative ways of meeting client needs that cost less are being explored. One such area is the use of advanced practice nurses (APNs) in various roles such as nurse practitioners, clinical nurse specialists, nurse midwives, and nurse anesthetists. Oxford Health Plans Inc., Norwalk, CT, an HMO, is currently employing nurse practitioners (NPs) to replace some primary physicians. These NPs are being paid what the physician would have been paid. If a problem arises that is outside of the NP's expertise, then the client is referred to a specialist.

There are both positive and negative aspects of care delivery being performed by APNs. The positive benefits are that the APN promotes health and wellness and identifies illness needs. The quality of the extended interaction between the client and the APN can lead to greater client satisfaction. If an HMO can achieve greater results at a lower cost, then the APN will earn a secure place in the health care system. The APN's assumption of liability for the care provided is the most problematic aspect of this specialty area. Questions raised about advance practice nursing by the medical community concern the length of study required for APN certification as compared to the educational preparation for physicians and the ability of APNs to recognize situations and needs for which the client should be referred to a specialist.

Of the many APN programs throughout the United States, there are 483 Nurse Practitioner programs (Romaine-Davis, 1997). All of these programs are on the graduate level and the requirements for a degree or certificate vary from institution to institution and program to program. The National Council of State Boards of Nursing and APN organizations are discussing the need for a second licensure examination for APNs. This will most likely lead to standardized APN curriculums that would require the same knowledge for an APN generic examination (Romaine-Davis, 1997).

For example, the University of Pennsylvania School of Nursing offers 17 advanced practice combination programs. They also have nine academic nursing practices that provide clinical sites for interdisciplinary education and research. Data collected at one of these sites showed that the nursing practice, compared to the HMO family practice physicians, "had lower overall costs per life, more primary care visits each year, an equal number of specialist visits, fewer hospital and emergency room visits and shorter hospital lengths-of-stay"(Lang, 1996).

It is clear that health care providers are closely watching the innovative moves taken by their colleagues. APNs are now very visible and are being provided with the opportunity to practice in ways that could dramatically change the health care delivery system and the contributions nurses will make to society.

IMAGE OF THE NURSING PROFESSION

The picture for nursing in general is not as clear as it is for advanced practice nursing. However, it is important to remember that nurses hold the health care system together. We are there caring for the client, listening and comforting. Unfortunately, many health care providers fail to recognize this contribution. Perhaps what is even sadder is that we do not appreciate who we are. Our profession has spent a great amount of time on the sensitive issue of professional status, with the result that deep divisions have been created from within nursing. The preference is that baccalaureate nurses be referred to as "professional" nurses and diploma and associate nurses be considered "technicians" or less than professional. Our energies have been spent on disagreeing among ourselves rather than in creating a vision for nursing. Meanwhile, many of our vital functions are being performed by crosstrained or unlicensed assistive personnel as we are relegated to the nurses' station with the paperwork. We need to appreciate the work that all of us do, with each playing a valuable role, and accept that when seen as a whole, the profession of nursing is making a tremendous contribution to health care.

LEGAL AND ETHICAL ISSUES

In community based practice, there may be times when you will be encouraged to practice nursing in a way that you believe is unethical, illegal, or both. For example, if a home care agency pursues a policy of making unnecessary visits so as to continue to receive payment, the nurse would need to collaborate with the agency through deliberately distorting nursing judgments and writing untruthful documentation. Despite such situations, if you keep your purpose and goals clearly in front of you, it will be easier to make decisions that are in line with both your ethical principles and the conditions of your licensure.

Because of the growth of health care expenditures on the federal level, many home care agencies have been established for monetary rather than for altruistic reasons. Home care costs are increasing at a rate of approximately 30% per year (Anders & McGinley, 1997). To decrease the cost of home care, changes will soon need to be made in the way these services are billed to Medicare. It is likely that a DRG system of managed care will be instituted to limit the number of visits that can be made to a client at home for a specific problem. Presently, the payment system is open ended, meaning that the number of visits that can be made for a specific condition is not limited. This practice encourages abuse of the system.

LIABILITY ISSUES

There are several factors that significantly increase the community based nurse's liability. One factor is the increased acute condition of the client in this setting. With all of its high technology, the hospital is moving into the home. The more complicated the technology, the greater the possibility of error on the part of the nurse, the client or family, and unskilled caregivers. The responsibility for teaching others how to care for the client at home falls on the nurse.

As the technological needs of the client in the community increase, there will be a shift within community based agencies in terms of hiring nurses with critical care backgrounds. Critical care nurses are usually "doers," and less likely to be intuitive or possess highly developed interpersonal skills. In this situation, it seems as if the technological or physical aspects of care could take precedence over the psychosocial aspects of that care. This trend could be particularly significant in the care of hospice clients.

The managed care system has placed tremendous pressure on agencies to produce effective and efficient results. This pressure is passed on to the nurses and places great demands on the nurse's time to meet deadlines of care and voluminous paperwork. Time constraints coupled with strict guidelines about the types and level of care delivered in an increasingly high-tech environment can easily lead to mistakes. If the caring of the nurse is not felt by the client due to being hurried or for other reasons and a mistake is made, the nurse has a greater chance of being involved in a lawsuit.

THE ROLE OF THE PHYSICIAN

We know that the hospital has truly moved into the home when physicians begin to make home visits, a practice that may soon become common. Six medical schools will each receive a $70,000 stipend to integrate home care into their curricula (Johnson, 1997). In the tradi-

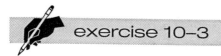

exercise 10–3

With the attitude of "anything is possible," create what you think home care of the near future will be like. Have fun.

....

....

....

....

....

tional medical practice model, the physician sees four to five patients in the time it takes to make one home visit. The greatest obstacle to revitalizing the physician-initiated house call is money because Medicare does not reimburse physicians for the full cost of a home visit or for travel. Once payors revise the reimbursement policies concerning home visits conducted by physicians and obtain approval of these policies by the medical profession, the home care curriculum model being developed for medical schools will be implemented.

This trend will lead to creative liaisons among health care professionals. Physicians, nurses, and other providers could make home visits together in high-tech vehicles. The possibilities are exciting and endless.

THE NATURE OF PARADIGMS

One characteristic of an emerging paradigm is that everyone goes back to zero (Barker, 1989). This means that all of the old rules no longer work. As a result, a different set of rules will be established to reflect the new paradigm. If these rules are unacceptable or unworkable, they will be discarded and replaced by still newer rules.

In the emerging health care paradigm, you can expect to see the new rules changing without warning. When trendsetters try something new and it does not seem to be working, changes will be made without notice. This approach, however, creates short-term instability. Eventually the rules will solidify. An example of the evolving nature of rules within emerging paradigms is seen in the care delivery system established by many HMOs. These organizations have made primary care physicians the gate-keepers to health care, meaning that these physicians not only make the decisions related to client referrals to specialists but also coordinate that care. This practice has caused dissatisfaction on the part of both physician and client.

On the other side of the spectrum is the service model developed by Oxford Health Plans, Inc. that places the care of clients who are experiencing chronic diseases and conditions such as cancer, heart disease, and prematurity under the supervision of specialists with the aim of minimizing or reducing the costs related to these disorders. This strategy does not return care to the old paradigm of unlimited access to services because a team of specialists will negotiate a fixed rate payment for each case. Clients will be asked about their progress after procedures and these responses will be included in the criteria for payment (Winslow, 1997).

This new way of coordinating client care will be continuously evaluated by Oxford, and other HMOs will be analyzing the results of this approach as well. If the system proves viable, chances are other companies will adopt it. If it proves to be ineffective, the rules will change again. You can expect these dramatic changes to occur until satisfactory solutions to numerous problems are found through trial and error.

The changes described above are taking place within the traditional or medical system. The characteristics of the medical paradigm, better known as the medical model, include a problem orientation, a focus on illness and disease rather than wellness, and treatment that consists of surgery and artificially produced medications. In this system, the patient is expected to conform to the prescribed medical regime with little or no input. The power is assumed to reside in the health care provider and in the system. This system automatically filters out opposing paradigms.

The other paradigm that has been gaining momentum in our culture has many names: holistic, wellness, alternative, or non-traditional. It developed outside of the traditional medical system. Its characteristics are the direct opposite of the medical paradigm and include: a focus on well-being; use of natural treatments; and an emphasis on personal power and self-responsibility.

The traditional medical system has dominated health care in our culture and has filtered other modalities from the mainstream of health care for many years. The nontraditional paradigm is influencing the general public to the extent that it is now becoming incorporated into the medical paradigm.

New paradigms usually replace the old. However, in this case, it is becoming evident that the two paradigms will co-exist. An example of this relationship can be found in the Oxford HMO. A client can choose to see either a primary physician or a certified alternative practitioner. The two paradigms are on equal footing in this case because the client does not need a referral from his primary physician to make an appointment with an alternative practitioner. The client is truly free to decide for himself. This process is dramatically different from physicians in the traditional medical system who make all the decisions about client referrals. If the Oxford HMO determines that its nontraditional focus is cost-effective, it is highly likely that more coalitions of this nature will emerge in the near future.

The media has made the concepts and various modalities of many nontraditional practices available to the general public. Alternative modalities have been the topic of discussion on radio and television programs and in newspaper and magazine articles. Most lay people are at least remotely familiar with the subject and many are curious about the implications of these new modalities. The demand for these interventions will explode once the public realizes they are readily available. This trend will increase the demand for more certified practitioners that, in turn, will lead to more career choices for members of our society and for nurses.

CAREER OPPORTUNITIES

The rapid and dramatic changes that are being experienced in the new health care paradigm create possibilities for a variety of employment opportunities and innovative business ventures. In this environment, your nursing skills will be an asset and, for many of these careers, licensure and your diploma or associate degree serve as sufficient preparation within these evolving careers.

When you decided to become a nurse, you put yourself through a very specific process. We are going to analyze exactly what you had to do in order to get as far as you have.

1. The first step in this process is to know exactly what you want. You set a goal that wraps around your dreams, decide how you are going to achieve that goal, and then pursue it with everything you have. A goal that will carry you through to the finish is one that you have a burning desire to accomplish. On the thinking level, this is something you want and on the feeling level, it is something you are going(!) to have.

2. Once you have set your goal, you must be prepared and willing to take whatever steps are required of you to achieve it. This includes actions that propel you forward. It is also just as important to stop doing what moves you further from your goal. The three actions that are capable of stopping you are: dwelling on the past, wasting time and energy on how difficult the process will be, and being afraid of making mistakes.

3. Maintain your belief, expectations and positive focus on your end result. Replace any negative thoughts with positive thoughts as you work toward your goal.

4. Be persistent. The feeling of being overwhelmed usually results from thinking about the whole picture and all that you have to accomplish in a short time. An effective way to handle this feeling is to focus on one small part at a time. This focus concentrates your energies on the task at hand and permits you to proceed.

5. Program your mind. You do this by becoming absorbed in your goal and the actions that move you in the desired direction. Positive thoughts lead to positive actions, thus creating a positive cycle.

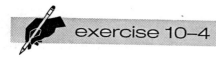

exercise 10–4

When you decided to become a nurse, you put yourself through the steps described above. Analyze exactly what you had to do in order to get as far as you have. With each step, identify what you did and how you did it.

1. ....
....
....
....
....

2. ....*grown*..
....
.................................*inward*...
.................................*upward*..
.................................*outward.*..

3. ....
....
....
....
....

4. ....
....
....
....
....

5. ....
....
....
....
....

The above steps can assist you with changes in your career goals. Stay open to opportunities. When you have an idea about developing possible career options, follow it through. Discuss your ideas with people who have done what you are considering. Those who have not attempted anything similar to what you want to do will often make statements that can discourage you. Those who have done it know exactly what you need and can be a tremendous resource to you.

There are many books, seminars, organizations, and other resources, such as the Internet, available to help you in exploring career opportunities. For example, if you are interested in self-employment, the National Nurses in Business (800-331-6534) is a non-profit organization that promotes the role of nurses in business. This is in addition to other self-employment resources available in your community.

The world is open to you, if you believe it. The combination of a dream, a goal and taking action will get you where you want to go. Enjoy!

REFERENCES

Anders, G. and McGinley, L. (1997). Medical morass: How do you tame a wild U.S. program?" *The Wall Street Journal,* Thursday, March 6, p 1.

Barker, J. (1989). *The Business of Paradigms.* (Video.) Discovering the Future Series. Burnsville MN: CHARTHOUSE International, (800-328-3789).

Johnson, L. (Associated Press.) (1997). House calls gain favor again among some doctors. *Star-Banner,* Monday, March 17.

Lang, N. (1996). Academic nursing practice: A case study of the university of Pennsylvania School of Nursing. *Penn Nursing* 1(1):18.

Romaine-Davis, A. (1997). *Advanced Practice Nurses.* Boston: Jones & Bartlett, p. 59.

Swansburg, R.C. (1997). *Budgeting and Financial Management for Nurse Managers.* Boston: Jones & Bartlett, pp. 123–167.

Winslow, R. (1997). Oxford to give more control to specialists. *The Wall Street Journal,* March 25, p. B1.

Index